EFOG Part 1

400 M...s, EMQs and

EFOG Part 1

400 MCQs, EMQs and SBAs

Sambit Mukhopadhyay MD DNB FRCOG MMed
Consultant Gynaecologist
Norfolk and Norwich University Hospital
Norwich, UK

Tahir A Mahmood CBE MD FRCPI FFSRH MBA FRCPE FRCOG
Consultant Obstetrician and Gynaecologist
Victoria Hospital,
Kirkcaldy, UK

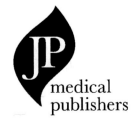

JP
medical
publishers

London • Panama City • New Delhi

© 2017 JP Medical Ltd.
Published by JP Medical Ltd
83 Victoria Street, London, SW1H 0HW, UK
Tel: +44 (0)20 3170 8910   Fax: +44 (0)20 3008 6180
Email: info@jpmedpub.com   Web: www.jpmedpub.com

ISBN: 978-1-909836-51-8

British Library Cataloguing in Publication Data
A catalogue record for this book is available from the British Library

Library of Congress Cataloging in Publication Data
A catalog record for this book is available from the Library of Congress

Commissioning Editor: Steffan Clements
Editorial Assistant: Adam Rajah
Design: Designers Collective Ltd

Preface

The European Board and College of Obstetrics and Gynaecology (EBCOG) introduced the European Fellowship in Obstetrics and Gynaecology (EFOG) examination for the purpose of determining whether the entrant possesses the knowledge required to deliver quality-assured care to women and their babies, as envisaged in the European curriculum of postgraduate training developed by the EBCOG.

The examination consists of two parts, and this book is a revision aid for Part 1. The 400 MCQs, EMQs and SBAs presented here cover every aspect of the syllabus, and the answers are in accordance with current practice. We have also included two practice papers, which if completed under timed conditions will provide a taste of the exam. In the Further Reading section we have referenced the latest studies in the field. The authors of the questions and explanations range from senior trainees to specialists actively involved in medical education, training and assessment.

Since the exam concentrates on applied knowledge, we recommend that candidates seek out as much clinical exposure as possible in the relevant areas. Candidates should be aware of the most recently published evidence for the management of women's health-related issues in obstetrics and gynaecology. Although there is no specific textbook recommended by the EBCOG, candidates should keep up to date with new developments in their specialty, and guidelines issued by the World Health Organization, the National Institute for Health and Care Excellence and equivalent European bodies.

We hope that this book builds your confidence by enabling you to identify your strengths and weaknesses, and that it gives you an insight into the structure of the examination. We believe that this practical guide will be invaluable to trainees all over the world who are preparing to take the EFOG examination.

Sambit Mukhopadhyay
Tahir A Mahmood
January 2017

Contents

Section C: Mock papers

Contributors

Ibrahim Alsharaydeh MRCOG
Senior Specialty Registrar
Obstetrics and Gynaecology Department
Royal Infirmary of Edinburgh,
Edinburgh, UK

Charlotte Cassis MBBS MA (Oxon)
Clinical Research Fellow
Norfolk and Norwich University Hospital,
Norwich, UK

Gomathy Gopal DFSRH MRCOG
Specialty Registrar
Obstetrics and Gynaecology Department
Ninewells Hospital,
Dundee, UK

Diana Marcus MBBS BSc (Hons) MRCOG MRCS
Specialty Trainee
Norwich and Norfolk University Hospital,
Norwich, UK
Clinical Research Fellow
Imperial College London,
London, UK

Asma Naqi MRCOG
Clinical Teaching Fellow
Obstetrics and Gynaecology Department
Norfolk and Norwich University Hospital,
Norwich UK

Mohamed A Otify MBBCh MSc Dip Gyn
Ultrasound MRCOG
Specialty Registrar
Royal Infirmary of Edinburgh,
Edinburgh, UK

Gautam Raje MBBS MD MRCOG
Consultant in Gynaecology
Norfolk and Norwich University Hospital,
Norwich, UK

Paul Simpson MA (Cantab) BMBS MRCOG
Specialty Registrar
Obstetrics and Gynaecology Department
Peterborough City Hospital,
Peterborough, UK

Medha M Sule FRCOG FRANZCOG MD MClined
Consultant in Gynaecology
Obstetrics and Gynaecology Department
Norfolk and Norwich University Hospital,
Norwich, UK
Honourary Senior Lecturer
University of East Anglia,
Norwich, UK

Martino Zacche MD
Clinical Fellow
Obstetrics and Gynaecology Department
Norfolk and Norwich University Hospital,
Norwich, UK

Acknowledgements

The editors are grateful to the contributors who have given up their valuable time, and also Dr Asma Naqi for organising the content of the book into various chapters.

Structure of the EFOG examination

Structure of the EFOG examination

The EFOG examination is divided into Part 1 and Part 2, the second of which may only be taken once the first has been passed:

- Part 1 – a knowledge-based assessment
- Part 2 – an objective structured clinical examination (OSCE)

Interested candidates should check the EBCOG website for up-to-date information and eligibility criteria for taking the fellowship examination.

The examination

Part 1 of the examination takes place at least once a year and coincides with the annual conference of the European Board of Obstetrics and Gynaecology. It consists of two papers covering obstetrics and gynaecology, each lasting 3 hours. The examination is taken online and the candidates should bring their own laptop computer. The examination is conducted over the course of one day.

The papers comprise a mixture of multiple choice questions (MCQs), single best answer questions (SBAs) and extended matching questions (EMQs). Each paper is marked out of 150, but the number and types of questions will vary as the EMQs are scored differently compared to MCQs and SBAs. The proportions of each type of question may also change because the examination structure is reviewed periodically. Both papers must be passed in order to pass the Part 1 examination.

Entrants who are successful in Part 1 should take Part 2 within a period of 3 years. Once this period has expired, or the entrant has failed to pass Part 2 within 3 years of passing Part 1, candidates must re-sit Part 1.

At the time of writing, the EBCOG does not have reciprocal arrangements with any other international examination bodies that allow entrants to claim exemption from Part 1.

Multiple choice questions

Each MCQ consists of a stem and a list of five options. The stem poses a problem or a statement, and the options are answers which may be true or false. Each option earns a point when answered correctly. There is no negative marking.

Single best answers

Each SBA assesses the application of knowledge in a particular clinical context and consists of a stem, a lead-in question and five answer options. The stem may include extended or ancillary material such as a vignette, a case study, a graph or a CTG output.

Candidates must select the single most appropriate answer from the options provided for that particular clinical context. Each SBA correctly answered will earn a point but the weightage of each point is different from MCQs.

There are four distractors surrounding the correct answer, and of these four there may be one or two that can be reasonably identified as incorrect. To choose the right answer from the remaining distractors, the candidate will need to reread the stem and then make a judgment as to which answer fits best.

Extending matching questions

An EMQ consists of several stems and a list of options. For each stem within the question, the candidate must select the correct answer from the list of options. The examination contains fewer EMQs than SBAs and MCQs but each questions carries higher weightage.

The candidate is advised to read the lead-in statement, formulate an answer in their head, and then look for the correct answer from the list of options. This will save time and avoid confusion.

As EMQs test the application of knowledge and the ability to synthesise knowledge, they take longer to answer than MCQs or SBAs. Therefore, it is advisable to answer these questions after completing MCQs and SBAs.

Part 2 – an objective structured clinical examination

Part 2 of the examination assesses a candidate's clinical skills in a variety of role-playing exercises. Examiners observe the candidate as they examine real or simulated patients at 10 stations. There is a rest station for reading a scientific article; another station for the evaluation of the article; two stations for basic technical skills (1 obstetrics and 1 gynaecology); two stations for complex technical skills (1 obstetrics and 1 gynaecology); two stations for knowledge integration and decision-making (1 obstetrics and 1 gynaecology); and two stations for communication skills. Candidates have two minutes of reading time and the examination is conducted in English. As with Part 1, the proportions of each type of station may not always be the same.

Section A

Obstetrics

Chapter 1

Preconception care

Questions: MCQs

Answer each stem 'True' or 'False'.

1. The following are examples of autosomal recessive conditions:
   - ✗A   Huntington's chorea
   - ✓B   Cystic fibrosis
   - ✗C   Marfan's syndrome
   - ✗D   Down's syndrome
   - ✗E   Haemophilia A

Questions: SBAs

For the following question, select the single best answer from the five options listed.

2. You are in the pre-pregnancy counselling clinic seeing a 19-year-old girl known to have asthma.

   How should it be managed?

   - A   The patient's medication should be modified once she is pregnant
   - ✓B   Management of an acute asthma attack should follow the same guidelines as in non-pregnant individuals
   - C   PEFR decreases in the third trimester of pregnancy
   - D   The patient should receive intravenous hydrocortisone in labour because of the increased risk of acute asthma in labour
   - E   Mild asthma in pregnancy may be associated with preeclampsia and intra-uterine growth restriction

Answers: MCQs

1. A False

    B True

    C False

    D False

    E False

    Huntington's chorea is an autosomal dominant condition expressed in heterozygotes. Cystic fibrosis is an example of an autosomal recessive condition. Marfan's syndrome is an example of an autosomal dominant condition. Down's syndrome is a chromosomal abnormality (as opposed to a genetic abnormality) where affected individuals carry an extra chromosome 21. Haemophilia A is an example of an X-linked recessive condition.

Answers: SBAs

2. B Management of an acute asthma attack should follow the same guidelines as in non-pregnant individuals

Many women still stop their asthma medication at the start of the pregnancy because of concerns regarding the safety profile of these drugs for the fetus. However, this should be discouraged and management of asthma in pregnancy should follow the British Thoracic Society guidelines as for the non-pregnant patient. PEFR is unchanged by pregnancy. Endogenous steroids in labour ensure that acute asthma attacks are very uncommon during labour and delivery. Intravenous hydrocortisone is only required in women taking > 7.5 mg prednisolone tablets for > 2 weeks prior to the onset of labour. A number of small studies have suggested an association of severe asthma with the development of pre-eclampsia, intra-uterine growth restriction (IUGR), preterm birth and low birth weight although most pregnancies are unaffected by the effects of asthma. Severe poorly controlled asthma resulting in episodes of maternal hypoxaemia could however give rise to such complications.

Chapter 2

Uncomplicated antenatal care

Questions: MCQs

Answer each stem 'True' or 'False'.

1. **The following vaccines can be administered during pregnancy:**
    - **A** MMR
    - **B** Influenza
    - **C** Hepatitis B
    - **D** Pneumococcus
    - **E** Herpes varicella zoster immunoglobulins

2. **With regards to the following maternal serum biomarkers:**
    - **A** Low levels of PAPP-A defined as less than 0.4–0.5 MoM have been associated with adverse fetal outcomes
    - **B** Low levels of free β-human chorionic gonadotrophin (β-hCG) (<0.5 MoM) in the 2nd trimester have been associated with low birth weight and increased risk of spontaneous miscarriage
    - **C** Elevated inhibin A in the first trimester (>2.0 MoM) has been associated with adverse outcomes such as gestational hypertension, pre-eclampsia, fetal growth restriction and fetal loss
    - **D** Reports have shown an association between placental abruption, placenta praevia, accreta, percreta and increta with elevated maternal serum α-feto protein
    - **E** First trimester levels of free β-hCG less than 5th percentile (0.41 MoM) had an odds ratio for spontaneous miscarriage > 1

Questions: SBAs

For the following question, select the single best answer from the five options listed.

3. A 25-year-old woman in her first pregnancy is seen at 40 weeks 5 days for a routine check. You are asked to counsel her about induction of labour.

   Which of the following statements is correct?

   A   Expectant management has been proven to be superior to routine induction of labour in preventing adverse outcomes

   B   Doppler velocimetry of the fetal circulation is a useful method to ascertain fetal wellbeing

   C   Induction of labour should be considered routinely prior to 41 weeks' gestation

   D   Cervical ripening prior to induce labour should be employed

   E   Continuous monitoring of the fetal heart is not recommended during labour

4. Which of the following lung function tests remains unchanged during pregnancy?

   A   pH

   B   Residual capacity

   C   Tidal volume

   D P_{CO_2}

   E   Bicarbonate

Answers: MCQs

1. A False

    B True

    C True

    D True

    E True

    All attenuated live vaccines are contraindicated during pregnancy and these include MMR (measles, mumps and rubella) and varicella zoster vaccine. Varicella zoster is a double-stranded DNA virus and is highly infectious. Varicella zoster immunoglobulins can be administered as soon as possible and can be given up to 10 days after significant exposure. The influenza and pneumoccocus vaccines contain previously virulent killed virus. The hepatitis B vaccine contains a protein sub unit which elicits an immune response from the surface of the virus.

2. A True

    B False

    C True

    D True

    E True

    Pregnancy-associated plasma protein-A (PAPP-A) is a protease for insulin-like growth factor (IGF) binding protein-4. Therefore, low levels of PAPP-A are associated with increased levels of binding protein, and subsequently low levels of free IGF. IGF controls the uptake and transport of glucose and amino acids in trophoblasts and plays a role in autocrine and paracrine invasion of trophoblasts into the decidua. Low levels of PAPP-A defined as less than 0.4–0.5 MoM have been associated with adverse fetal outcomes, especially those that may be linked to abnormal trophoblastic invasion.

    In the first trimester, low levels of free β-human chorionic gonadotrophin (β-hCG) (< 0.5 MoM) have been associated with low birthweight and increased risk of spontaneous miscarriage. First trimester elevations in free β-hCG have not been associated with any adverse obstetric outcome. The converse holds true for the second trimester. Low levels of β-hCG have not been linked to adverse outcomes, however, elevated β-hCG (>2–4 MoM) has been associated with multiple adverse outcomes. Elevated inhibin A in the second trimester (>2.0 MoM) has been associated with adverse outcomes such as gestational hypertension, pre-eclampsia, fetal growth restriction and fetal loss.

Answers: SBAs

3. D Cervical ripening prior to induce labour should be employed

In spite of several studies, it is still not clear whether expectant management is superior to routine induction of labour for preventing adverse outcomes in prolonged pregnancy. The efficacy of Doppler velocimetry of the fetal or uteroplacental circulation in predicting outcome has not been proven. At present it is not recommended in the monitoring of a post-term pregnancy. There is no place for routine induction of labour prior to 41 weeks' gestation. It may in fact increase the risk of failed induction and rate of caesarean delivery. Induction of labour prior to 41 weeks' gestation should only be considered in the presence of risk factors. There is no evidence to indicate that induction prior to 41 weeks is of any benefit to either the mother or the fetus. The findings of large, placebo-controlled trials support the use of cervical ripening agents to reduce the rate of caesarean delivery due to failed induction. The risks associated with the use of such agents, e.g. uterine hyperstimulation or non-reassuring fetal heart rate patterns, should however be remembered. The patient's history needs to be carefully considered; for instance if the woman had a previous caesarean delivery, she is at an increased risk of scar rupture. Due to an increased incidence of meconium staining of liquor and non-reassuring fetal heart rate patterns in prolonged pregnancies, continuous monitoring of the fetal heart is recommended.

4. A pH

During pregnancy, residual volume decreases, tidal volume increases as in minute ventilation, pCO_2 falls and pH remains unchanged.

Chapter 3

Complicated antenatal care

Questions: MCQs

Answer each stem 'True' or 'False'.

1. The following factors are associated with increased risk of breast cancer:
   - A   Multiparity
   - B   Late first pregnancy
   - C   Early menarche
   - D   Pre-eclampsia
   - E   Bottle feeding

2. Regarding breast cancer during pregnancy:
   - A   Breast cancer affects 1 in 1000 pregnant women 1 : 3000
   - B   *BRCA1* and *BRCA2* mutations confer an equal risk of development of breast cancer
   - C   Tamoxifen cannot be given during pregnancy
   - D   Chemotherapy should be avoided during the second trimester
   - E   Radiotherapy following surgery during pregnancy should be delayed until delivery

3. Regarding the diagnosis and management of pre-term pre-labour rupture of membranes:
   - A   Abnormal biophysical profile has a 90% positive predictive value for chorioamnionitis
   - B   Doppler studies have a >70% sensitivity to diagnose chorioamnionitis
   - C   Treatment with co-amoxiclav (augmentin) reduces the risk of necrotising enterocolitis
   - D   Erythromycin reduces the incidence of delivery within 48 hours
   - E   Antenatal steroids should not be administered if chorioamnionitis is suspected

4. Regarding bacterial sepsis in pregnancy:
   - A   Severe sepsis with acute organ dysfunction is associated with 5–10% mortality 20 – 40 rate
   - B   Urinary tract infection and chorioamnionitis are the most common infections associated with septic shock

    C   Severe infection is associated with preterm labour
    D   Signs and symptoms of sepsis are more distinctive in pregnancy
    E   Progression of sepsis may be more rapid

5.   **Regarding bacterial sepsis following pregnancy:**
    A   Contact with birthing animals is associated with *Chlamydia pssittaci* infection
    B   Contact with aborting sheep is associated with Q fever (*Coxiella burnetti*) infection
    C   Ingestion of milk products is associated with *Listeria* infection
    D   Healthcare workers who have been exposed to respiratory secretions of women with group A streptococcal infection should be considered for antibiotic prophylaxis
    E   High dose IVIG (intravenous immunoglobulin) is effective against endotoxic shock

6.   **Regarding varicella zoster infection in pregnancy:**
    A   A planned delivery should be avoided for at least 5 days after the onset of the maternal rash
    B   Intravenous acyclovir should be given to all pregnant women with severe chickenpox
    C   The risk of spontaneous miscarriage is increased if chickenpox occurs in the first trimester
    D   There is a significant risk of varicella infection of the newborn, if maternal infection occurs in the last 4 weeks of a woman's pregnancy.
    E   There is a small risk of fetal varicella syndrome (FVS), if the pregnant woman shows serological conversion in the second 28 weeks of pregnancy. *1st*

7.   **Regarding breast cancer and pregnancy:**
    A   Anthracyline regimens are safe in second trimester
    B   Breast reconstruction surgery can safely be carried out in pregnancy
    C   Echocardiography should be performed during pregnancy in women at risk to detect cardiomyopathy
    D   Trastuzumab can be used in pregnancy *& Tamoxifin C-Indicate*
    E   Women should wait at least 2 years after treatment before contemplating pregnancy

Questions: SBAs

For each question, select the single best answer from the five options listed.

8. A healthy 24-year-old woman in her first pregnancy is admitted at 29 weeks' gestation with confirmed preterm, prelabour rupture of membranes.

    What is the next course of action?

    A   Consider delivery as the fetus is at significant risk of pulmonary hypoplasia
    B   Immediate delivery is indicated to reduce the risk of infection
    C   Caesarean section is indicated to avoid fetal compromise and trauma
    D   Administer co-amoxiclav
    E   Inform neonatology registrar

9. Induction of labour is recommended beyond 41 weeks' gestation.

    Of the following the most important reason for inducing labour beyond 41 weeks is:

    A   To reduce the incidence of neonatal seizures
    B   To reduce meconium staining of the liquor
    C   To reduce perinatal mortality
    D   To reduce the instrumental delivery rates
    E   To reduce the caesarean section rates

10. Of the following vaccines, which one should be avoided during pregnancy?

    A   Tetanus vaccine
    B   Diphtheria vaccine
    C   Flu vaccine
    D   Measles vaccine
    E   Pertussis vaccine

11. Maternal intravenous immunoglobulin (IVIG) is now the first line treatment for one of the following:

    A   Prevention of fetal congenital heart block
    B   Fetal alloimmune thrombocytopenia
    C   Rhesus D isoimmunisation
    D   Prevention of fetal virilisation in congenital adrenal hyperplasia
    E   Fetal parvovirus infection

12. With regards to parvovirus, which of the following is correct?

    A   80% of women of child-bearing age are immune
    B   Women with a presumed parvovirus rash should stay away from antenatal clinics and other pregnant women
    C   It can cause a maternal aplastic crisis
    D   1 in 4 fetuses will become hydropic
    E   Hydropic fetuses receiving steroid injections have normal outcomes if they survive to term

13. With regards to cytomegalovirus (CMV) infection in pregnancy, which of the following is correct?

A   Amniocentesis at 18 weeks is a reliable tool for investigating vertical transmission

B   Amniocentesis should be delayed for 6 weeks following the maternal infection

C   1 in 4 fetuses will be damaged following a proven fetal CMV infection

D   10% of infected fetuses will show clinical sequelae at birth

E   90% of babies born with evidence of CMV will have long-term neurological damage

Questions: EMQs

Question 14 – 18

Option for Questions 14 – 18:

A Abruption of placenta
B Accidental haemorrhage
C Unexplained haemorrhage
D In labour
E Intrauterine death

F Placenta accreta
G Placenta praevia
H Preterm labour
I Primary postpartum haemorrhage
J Secondary postpartum haemorrhage

For each case described below, choose the single most appropriate diagnosis from above list of options. Each option may be used once, more than once, or not at all.

14. A 23-year-old woman is 40 weeks pregnant. She presents to hospital with a history of reduced fetal movements. She says that abdominal contractions are coming every few minutes and she has been having a blood-stained discharge per vagina. On vaginal examination the cervix is 5 cm dilated, with cephalic presentation and station is +1.

15. A 31-year-old primigravida, who is 30 weeks pregnant, presents to the emergency department with absent fetal movements. She also complains of severe headache, heartburn and blurring of vision for the last few days. On examination, her blood pressure is 170/110 mmHg, a urine dipstick shows ++++ protein, and abdominally her uterus is hard and tender with no visible signs of fetal movement per abdomen.

16. A 32-year-old pregnant woman in her first pregnancy at 36/40 weeks by date presents to the labour ward with a history of painless significant vaginal bleeding after sexual intercourse. On examination the abdomen is soft and not tender. The fetus is presenting by the head and is 5/5th palpable above the symphysis pubis. Cardiotocography (CTG) is normal.

17. A 26-year-old primigravida, who is 40 weeks pregnant, presents to the labour ward with a history of constant abdominal pain for the last few hours. She also gives a history of having lost a cupful of fresh blood per vagina before the pain started. Abdominal examination shows an irritable uterus. CTG was normal.

18. A 35-year-old woman had a vaginal delivery 7 days ago. She presents to her general practitioner with a history of a foul-smelling discharge per vagina. She also gives a history of passing blood clots per vagina for the last 24 hours. On examination her blood pressure is 90/40 mmHg, her pulse is 110 beats/minute and her temperature is 38°C. On abdominal examination uterus is tender on palpation and the uterine fundus is 2 cm above the umbilicus. Speculum examination reveals clots in the vagina.

Question 19 – 22

Options for Questions 19 – 22:

A	Mesenteric vein thrombosis	J	Acute fatty liver
B	Pancreatitis	K	Severe constipation
C	Appendicitis	L	Abruption
D	Ureteric colic	M	Preterm labour
E	Pyelonephritis	N	Urinary retention
F	Torsion of an ovarian cyst	O	Sickle cell crisis
G	Pre-eclampsia	P	Crohn's disease
H	Red degeneration	Q	Ulcerative colitis
I	HELLP (haemolytic anaemia, elevated liver enzymes and low platelet count) syndrome	R	None of the above

For each case described below, choose the single most appropriate diagnosis from the above list of options. Each option may be used once, more than once, or not at all.

19. A 20-year-old woman in her first pregnancy is admitted with severe abdominal pain at 30 weeks' gestation. She describes the pain to be radiating from her back to her groin. She was treated for an episode of fever with chills a month ago by her general practitioner. Urinalysis showed leucocytes and blood. Her blood test results are as follows: haemoglobin 97 g/L, white blood cell count 19 × 10^9/L, platelets 180 × 10^9/L, uric acid 0.35 mmol/L, amylase 150 IU/L, aspartate aminotransferase (AST) 22 IU/L and alanine aminotransferase (ALT) 27 IU/L.

20. A 29-year-old woman attends the day assessment unit with abdominal pain. She is 30 weeks pregnant in her fourth pregnancy. She also gives a history of nausea and vomiting since morning. There is no history of tightening, or bleeding per vaginum. She drinks 24 units of alcohol a week. Her blood pressure is 135/85 mmHg and pulse is 105 beats/minute. Urine analysis is negative. Her blood results are: haemoglobin 125 g/L, white blood cell count 13 × 10^9/L, C-reactive protein (CRP) 210 mg/L, AST 42 IU/L, gamma-glutamyl transferase (GGT) 55 IU/L, alkaline phosphatase (ALP) 250 IU/L, amylase 700 IU/L and bilirubin 32 μmol/L.

21. A 29-year-old woman in her first pregnancy presents to accident and emergency at 34 weeks' gestation with a history of acute abdominal pain. She is agitated, confused, and complains of headache and severe nausea. There is no history of uterine tightening or bleeding per vaginum. Her blood pressure is 135/80 mmHg and urinalysis shows 3+ protein. Her initial blood results are: haemoglobin 115 g/L, white blood cell count 9 × 10^9/L, CRP 150 mg/L, AST 110 IU/L, GGT 87 IU/L, ALP 660 IU/L, bilirubin 427.60 μmol/L, amylase 65 IU/L and serum albumin 20 g/dL.

22. A 33-year-old primigravid woman presents with lower abdominal pain at 16 weeks' gestation. There is no history of vaginal bleeding or dysuria. She had an episode of vomiting in the morning. On examination her temperature is 37.9°C. There is tenderness in her lower abdomen, particularly the right lower quadrant. Vaginal examination reveals a closed cervix with no bleeding. Blood results are: haemoglobin 135 g/L, white blood cell count 17 × 10^9/L, CRP 740 mg/L, AST 32 U/L, GGT 19 IU/L, ALP 155 IU/L, bilirubin 20 μmol/L, amylase 55 IU and serum albumin 280 g/L.

Question 23 – 27

Options for Questions 23 – 27:

A   Prescribe oral acyclovir for 7 days
B   Warn to stay away from hospital because of the infectious nature of her condition
C   Refer to hospital
D   Requires an immediate caesarean section under epidural anaesthesia to avoid the theoretical transmission of the virus from skin lesions to CNS in a spinal anaesthesia
E   Administer varicella zoster immunoglobulin (VZIG) as soon as possible
F   Prescribe a 10-day course of prophylaxis with zanamivir or oseltamivir as soon as possible
G   Investigate with sputum culture and chest radiograph
H   Treat empirically for pneumonia, avoiding chest radiograph but with supportive measures including oxygen administration and rehydration and oral antibiotic therapy
I   Institute supportive treatment and intravenous acyclovir

For each case described below, choose the single most appropriate course of action from the above list of options. Each option may be used once, more than once, or not at all.

23. A 28-year-old woman presents at 28 weeks gestation with a 3-day history of a rash and chesty cough and a history of recent exposure to chickenpox. She smokes 20 cigarettes per day.

24. A 29-year-old pregnant woman develops a fever, cough and sore throat 2 days after arrival in the UK from a visit to Zambia.

25. A 19-year-old woman presents to the emergency department with breathlessness, fever and a cough productive of green sputum. On admission she tests positive for pregnancy.

26. A 28-year-old woman presents unwell with symptoms and signs of varicella infection, difficulty breathing and fever at 39 weeks' gestation.

27. A 25-year-old woman is exposed to chickenpox at 16 weeks' gestation. A serum test sent 9 days after exposure is negative for VZIG.

Answers: MCQs

1. A False

    B True

    C True

    D False

    E True

    Risk factors for the development of breast cancer include nulliparity, early menarche, late first pregnancy, BRCA1 and BRCA2 mutations. The risk of breast cancer is also increased after pregnancy for a maximum of 3–4 years. Protective factors include higher parity, pre-eclampsia and breast feeding. The protective effect of breast feeding is related to duration of lactation.

2. A False

    B False

    C True

    D True

    E True

    Breast cancer affects about 1 in 3000 pregnant women. Mutations in the BRCA1 and BRCA2 genes have different risk profiles for development of breast cancer. Surgical excision can be undertaken at any stage in pregnancy but reconstructive surgery should be delayed till delivery. Chemotherapy should be avoided in the first trimester and Tamoxifen is contra-indicated during pregnancy. Radiotherapy should be delayed until delivery unless it is life-saving.

3. A False

    B False

    C False

    D True

    E False

    The positive predictive value of abnormal biophysical profile in predicting chorio-amnionitis ranges from 30–80%. Doppler studies have not shown to be very useful and their sensitivity is around 20–40%. Treatment with co-amoxyclav has a strong association with development of necrotising enterocolitis. Erythromycin reduces the incidence of delivery within 48 hours. Antenatal steroids should be administered even if chorioamnionitis is suspected as the risk of respiratory distress syndrome, necrotising enterocolitis and intraventricular haemorrhage is reduced.

4. A False

    B True

    C True

    D False

    E True

    Severe sepsis with acute organ dysfunction is associated with 20–40% mortality rate. Due to physiological and hormonal changes in pregnancy, signs and symptoms of sepsis are less distinctive. Intravenous immunoglobulin (IVIG) is recommended for severe invasive streptococcal infection when antibiotic treatment has failed.

5. A False

    B False

    C True

    D True

    E False

    Contact with birthing animals is associated with Q fever (*Coxilla burnetti*). Contact with aborting sheep is associated with *Chlamydia psittaci*. Antibiotic treatment is required if the mother, baby or both are infected.

6. A False

    B True

    C False

    D True

    E False

    A planned delivery should normally be avoided for at least 7 days after the onset of the maternal rash to allow for the passive transfer of antibodies from mother to child, provided that continuing the pregnancy does not pose any additional risks to the mother or baby. Spontaneous miscarriage does not appear to be increased if chickenpox occurs in the first trimester. If the pregnant woman develops varicella or shows serological conversion in the first 28 weeks of pregnancy, she has a small risk of fetal varicella syndrome and she should be informed of the implications.

7. A True

    B False

    C True

    D False

    E True

Breast reconstruction should be delayed to avoid prolonged anaesthesia and to allow optimal symmetrisation of the breasts after delivery. These women may have received adjuvant chemotherapy with anthracyclines (doxorubicin, epirubicin), which can cause cumulative dose-dependent left ventricular dysfunction and, rarely, cardiomyopathy.

Although cardiac complications during pregnancy are rare in cancer survivors, echocardiography should be performed during pregnancy in women at risk to detect cardiomyopathy through resting left ventricular ejection fraction or echocardiographic fractional shortening. Systemic chemotherapy is contraindicated in the first trimester because of a high rate of fetal abnormality, but is safe from the second trimester and should be offered according to protocols defined by the risk of breast cancer relapse and mortality. Anthracyclines regimens are safe; there are fewer data on taxanes. Tamoxifen and trastuzumab are contraindicated in pregnancy and should not be used.

Answers: SBAs

8. E Inform neonatology registrar

Pulmonary hypoplasia is likely to happen when premature rupture of membranes (PROM) occurs for more than 7 days before 26 weeks. After that gestation it is very unlikely. The results of the Oracle trial showed that giving the use of co-amoxiclav (augmentin) was associated with a significantly higher rate of neonatal necrotising enterocolitis. Caesarean section is an option only when woman in labour. Delivery is indicated at 34 weeks for pregnant women Group B *Streptococcus* (GBS) carrier with no signs of chorioamnionitis. Preterm PROM increased the risk of preterm labour, and neonatology unit needed to be notified and ready to take the baby if delivered preterm.

9. C To reduce perinatal mortality

Induction of labour (IOL) at 41+ weeks has the following effects:

- Reduces perinatal mortality by 1 baby per 500 inductions; the number needed to treat is 500 (the main reason behind offering IOL beyond 41 weeks)
- Reduces the caesarean section rate
- Reduces meconium staining
- Does not result in a change in the instrumental delivery rate

10. D Measles vaccine

As a general rule, live vaccines, either viral or bacterial, should not be given during pregnancy. Tetanus, diphtheria and pertussis vaccines are toxoids, therefore their use in pregnancy is permitted. Studies have shown that the flu vaccine is safe during any stage of pregnancy, from the first few weeks up to the expected due date. Measles vaccines contain live attenuated virus, and should be avoided in pregnancy.

11. B Fetal alloimmune thrombocytopenia

Fetal and neonatal alloimmune thrombocytopenia is no longer managed by serial intrauterine platelet transfusions, which are hazardous and no more effective at preventing fetal intracranial bleeding than maternal intravenous immunoglobulin (IVIG) administration. Although severe cases of rhesus D isoimmunisation have been treated in a similar way with IVIG, this is not first line and is only employed when the first transfusion is anticipated to be very early in the pregnancy (at < 24 weeks' gestation). A trial using IVIG to prevent congenital heart block in the offspring of women carrying anti-Ro and anti-La antibodies did not show a convincing benefit. However, the evidence supporting high-dose steroid regimes is also poor. The Corticosteroids are used to help prevent virilisation of a female fetus in congenital adrenal hyperplasia, but IVIG is not used. IVIG is not used to treat parvovirus infections either; these may require an intrauterine transfusion.

12. C It can cause a maternal aplastic crisis

Approximately 50% of women are parvovirus non-immune and remain vulnerable to an infection during pregnancy. Parvovirus is only infectious before the rash occurs so it is safe for women to be assessed in a maternity department when a parvovirus rash is expected. Aplastic crises causing anaemia may occur in the fetus but also in the woman herself if she has other underlying causes of red cell haemolysis such as spherocytosis, pyruvate kinase deficiency and sickle cell disease. The risk of hydrops is probably no greater than 1 in 10 when infection occurs during pregnancy. Even when the fetus is severely hydropic and extremely anaemic, the long term outcome is usually good if the fetus survives the intrauterine transfusion, of which only one is usually required.

13. A Amniocentesis at 18 weeks is a reliable tool for investigating vertical transmission

Cytomegalovirus (CMV) DNA only appears in amniotic fluid when the fetus begins to pass considerable volumes of urine, which is usually thought to occur beyond 20–22 weeks' gestation.

There is a 6 week latency period between maternal infection and the excretion of CMV in fetal urine. False negatives are possible therefore if timing is inappropriate. 10% of infected fetuses will show clinical sequelae at birth, however another 10–15% will be found to be affected at some later point, principally by sensorineural deafness.

90% of those affected at birth will develop a long-term neurological handicap.

Answers: EMQ

14. D In labour

In pregnancy and labour many women present with symptoms that could indicate a serious condition, but have no problems. The history of diminished fetal movements is not unusual late in pregnancy and particularly with the onset of labour. It should be investigated by a cardiotocography, but on its own does not imply a problem. Also, many women have a bloody 'show' in labour.

15. A Abruption of placenta

The symptoms indicate severe pre-eclampsia leading to placental abruption.

16. G Placenta praevia

Painless vaginal bleeding with a high head at term in a primigravida is placenta praevia till proven otherwise.

17. A Abruption of placenta

This is the most likely diagnosis from the clinical picture.

18. J Secondary postpartum haemorrhage (PPH)

Primary postpartum haemorrhage is bleeding from the genital tract in excess of 500 mL in the first 24 hours after delivery. Secondary PPH (as in this case) is any significant bleeding from the genital tract between 24 hours and 6 weeks after birth. The commonest cause is infection.

19. E Pyelonephritis

Pyelonephritis is common in pregnancy due to physiological changes in the urinary tract during pregnancy.

20. B Pancreatitis

Gallstones and alcoholism are the common causes of acute pancreatitis, and treatment is intensive supportive therapy.

21. J Acute fatty liver

Acute fatty liver is rare in pregnancy but the prognosis is poor. It usually occurs in patients with pre-eclampsia.

22. C Appendicitis

Appendicitis commonly presents in the early second trimester in young mothers. The classical signs might be absent in pregnancy.

23. C Refer to hospital

Women who develop chickenpox in the latter half of pregnancy are at increased risk of developing pneumonia and other complications. Oral acyclovir reduces the duration of fever and symptoms only when commenced within 24 hours of developing the rash. It is of no benefit if commenced after 24 hours. The development of chest symptoms is an indication for referral to hospital. The Royal College of Obstetricians and Gynaecologists guidelines also recommend considering hospital assessment in women with chickenpox who smoke even in the absence of complications.

24. G Investigate with sputum culture and chest radiograph

The incidence of tuberculosis (TB) worldwide is rising, in part due to susceptibility to TB of HIV-infected patients and in the UK is more prevalent amongst Asian and African immigrants. The diagnosis of TB is confirmed with sputum examination for acid-fast bacilli (Ziehl–Neelsen stain).

25. G Investigate with sputum culture and chest radiograph

Reluctance to perform a chest X-ray in pregnancy can delay a diagnosis. Ionising radiation from a chest X-ray is approximately 0.2 rad (< 1/20th of maximum recommended exposure in pregnancy) and abdominal shielding will reduce fetal exposure further.

26. I Institute supportive treatment and intravenous acyclovir

Delivery during a viraemic period is hazardous with maternal risks of bleeding, thrombocytopenia, disseminated intravascular coagulation and hepatitis. Aim to avoid delivery and provide supportive treatment and intravenous acyclovir, however delivery may be required in women to facilitate assisted ventilation in cases complicated by respiratory failure.

27. E Administer varicella zoster immunoglobulin (VZIG) as soon as possible

All nonimmune pregnant women exposed to varicella should be given zoster immunoglobulin (ZIG) as soon as possible. VZIG is effective when given up to 10 days after contact, and administration can be delayed until serology results are known.

Chapter 4

Maternal disorders in pregnancy

Questions: MCQs

Answer each stem 'True' or 'False'.

1. **Regarding the effect of pregnancy on cardiac disease:**
    - ✗A Pregnancy decreases the incidence of cardiac arrhythmia due to hormonal changes
    - B Pregnancy in women who have had mechanical valve replacement is associated with a 45% incidence of thrombotic episodes
    - C Antibiotic prophylaxis should be given during labour and delivery for all women with valvular lesions except mitral valve prolapse without regurgitation
    - ✗D There is a 70% mortality rate with New York Heart Association class III or IV 7%.
    - E The overall risk of inheriting polygenic cardiac disease is quoted at 3–5%

2. **Regarding thyroid disease in pregnancy:**
    - ✗A Clinical disease activity follows the titre of thyroid-stimulating hormone (TSH) receptor stimulating antibodies, which falls in the first trimester and ↑ puerperium and rise in the second and third trimester. ↓
    - B Propylthiouracil causes aplasia cutis congenita *Carbamizole*
    - C Most pregnant women will need to increase their dose in the puerperium to avoid a relapse of hyperthyroidism
    - D The risk of fetal Graves' disease after 20 weeks is inversely proportional to the mother's TSH receptor stimulating antibodies titre
    - E Fetal Graves' disease can cause craniosynostosis and associated intellectual impairment

3. **In women with cystic fibrosis who present in pregnancy:**
    - A A course of oral antibiotics is often required should the patient develop any chest infection ↳
    - B Breastfeeding women with cystic fibrosis may find it difficult to breastfeed exclusively
    - C If the partner does not carry any of the common gene mutations for cystic fibrosis, the risk of having an affected child is 1:250
    - D Oral glucose tolerance should be done not before 24–28 weeks
    - E If regional anaesthesia is used, an epidural catheter can be left in place to assist with pain relief and postoperative chest physiotherapy

4.   **In prolactinomas:**

A   During pregnancy, the risk of tumour enlargement may occur in 3% of those with macroadenomas 32%

B   For women who remain symptom-free throughout pregnancy, serum prolactin should be measured 2 months after delivery

C   If the enlarged tumour does not respond to cabergoline therapy, transsphenoidal surgery in the second trimester can be considered

D   Pregnancy induces remission of hyperprolactinemia in two-thirds of women after continuation of dopamine agonist

E   Serial MRI examinations or visual field testing during pregnancy is required

5.   **Regarding pregnant women with epilepsy**

A   Oral vitamin K should be given to all patients on enzyme-inducing anti-epileptic drugs (AEDs) to prevent haemorrhagic disease of the newborn

B   Pethidine can be safely used in women with epilepsy in labour

C   Therapeutic drug monitoring reduces risk of seizure deterioration

D   There is an increased risk of depression in women with epilepsy

E   There is enough evidence to suggest giving double the dose of steroids in women with epilepsy presenting with preterm labour

6.   **Regarding pregnancy after a renal transplant**

A   Renal transplant improves the fertility rate to > 1:50

B   Globular filtration rates do not increase during pregnancy

C   There is increased risk of developing hypertension

D   Cyclosporins should be stopped after the 1st trimester

E   Fetal growth is usually optimal in women with stable renal transplant

Questions: SBAs

For each question, select the single best answer from the five options listed.

7. A 29-year-old woman with bipolar affective disorder finds herself pregnant for the first time.

    With regards to her management all of the following statements are true except:

    A   Women taking lithium should be changed immediately to an alternative upon becoming pregnant
    B   The risk of perinatal relapse is approximately 1 in 2
    C   Breastfeeding is not recommended for women taking lithium
    D   Neonatal lithium toxicity can lead to neonatal hypothyroidism and diabetes insipidus
    E   Postpartum new-onset disorders of this kind usually present within the first week following birth

8. A general practitioner has asked your advice about a patient with a severe migraine. He is concerned about the safety of a drug in pregnancy. The patient has a longstanding history of migraine and is currently 20 weeks pregnant.

    Of the following drugs which one should be avoided in the management of migraines in this patient?

    A   Sumatriptan
    B   Amitriptyline
    C   Ibuprofen
    D   Dihydrocodeine
    E   Verapamil

Questions: EMQs

Questions 9 – 10

Option list for Questions 9 – 10

A	Amniotic fluid embolism	I	Placental abruption
B	Peripartum cardiomyopathy	J	Placenta praevia
C	Chest infection	K	Pulmonary embolism
D	Cerebro-vascular accident	L	Pulmonary hypertension
E	Endocarditis	M	Sepsis
F	Haemorrhage	N	Substance misuse
G	HELLP syndrome	O	Thromboembolism
H	Myocardial infarction		

For each case described below, choose the single most likely cause of maternal death from the above list of options. Each option may be used once, more than once, or not at all.

9. A previously healthy 24-year-old primigravida presents at 34 weeks of pregnancy feeling unwell and tired. Her brother died unexpectedly some years ago, aged 25 years. Her chest X-ray shows an enlarged heart. While being admitted she develops increasing shortness of breath and dies despite intensive resuscitation.

10. A 26-year-old woman at 30 weeks' gestation in her fifth pregnancy presents to the emergency department with breathlessness and displays severe anxiety. She has complained of left-sided pelvic pain for a week. While being assessed she collapses. It is not possible to resuscitate her.

Questions 11–15

Option list for Questions 11–15

A	HELLP syndrome	G	Neonatal alloimmune
B	Thrombotic thrombocytopenic		thrombocytopenia
	purpura	H	Disseminated intravascular
C	Von Willebrand's disease type IIB		coagulation
D	Acute fatty liver of pregnancy	I	Haemolytic uraemic syndrome
E	Gestational thrombocytopenia	J	Viral infection
F	Idiopathic thrombocytopenic purpura		

For each case described below, choose the single most appropriate diagnosis from above list of options. Each option may be used once, more than once, or not at all.

11. A 25-year-old pregnant woman in her first pregnancy presents at 26 weeks with hemiplegia, paresthesias, visual disturbance, fatigue and dark urine. She has an ADAMTs-13 protein deficiency and suffers from microangiopathic haemolytic anaemia and purpura.

12. A 19-year-old pregnant woman is in her first pregnancy. Recently she went on trip to a petting zoo. She presents at 16 weeks with nausea and vomiting, and haemorrhagic diarrhoea. A few hours after admission to hospital she becomes irritable, oliguric and has a self-limiting seizure. Her blood picture shows mildly elevated bilirubin, reticulocytosis, low haemoglobin and platelets, and grossly abnormal renal function tests.

13. A 32-year-old pregnant woman is in her first pregnancy. She presents at 37 weeks with sudden onset severe abdominal pain and vaginal bleeding. Intrauterine fetal death is confirmed on admission. One hour after admission to the labour ward, vaginal bleeding becomes severe, and she becomes unstable. An urgent caesarean section is performed, which is complicated with atonic uterus and she loses 7.5 L of blood. A caesarean hysterectomy is eventually performed to control bleeding. She is given 32 units of different blood products.

14. A 32-year-old pregnant woman in her first pregnancy presents at 35 weeks' gestation with malaise, nausea and vomiting and severe epigastric pain. Her clinical condition deteriorates within a few hours after admission. Her blood results show hypoglycaemia, hyperuricaemia, raised creatinine, urea and grossly abnormal liver function tests.

15. An 18-year-old pregnant woman in her first pregnancy presents at 36 weeks to obstetric triage with headache, blurring vision and swelling of her feet. Her blood pressure is 180/110 mmHg with +++ protein in her urine. Her blood investigations show haemoglobin 99 g/L, platelets 80×10^9/L, alanine aminotransferase (ALT) 265 IU/L, urea 6.7 mmol/L, creatinine 46 μmol/L and uric acid 580 μmol/L.

Questions 16 – 19

Option list for Questions 16 – 19

A	Postpartum cardiomyopathy	I	Cervical trauma
B	Thromboembolism	J	Fat embolism
C	Amniotic fluid embolism	K	Anaphylaxis
D	Vaginal tear	L	Postpartum collapse
E	Uterine inversion	M	Torsion of an ovarian cyst
F	Atonic postpartum haemorrhage	N	Thrombosis of the sagittal sinus
G	Eclampsia	O	Subarachnoid haemorrhage
H	Epilepsy		

For each description below, choose the single most appropriate diagnosis from the above list of options. Each option may be used once, more than once, or not at all.

16. A 36-year-old woman in her first pregnancy has had a low-cavity forceps delivery for prolonged second stage under spinal anaesthesia. After delivery she experiences excessive vaginal bleeding. On examination she is noted to have excessive blood loss and appeared pale. Her pulse is 120 beats/minute and blood pressure 110/60 mmHg. Abdominal examination reveals a well-contracted uterus. Examination of the placenta confirms it to be complete.

17. A 28-year-old woman in her third pregnancy has been admitted to the hospital with severe abdominal pain. She had been evaluated for a suspicious adnexal mass during the antenatal period. She collapses in the bathroom on the first postnatal day.

18. A 34-year-old who is para 4 has a quick labour. The baby weighs 4.8 kg. Examination of the placenta is complete. On examination she is pale and clammy. The maternal pulse demonstrates a tachycardia of 100 beats/minute and her blood pressure is 90/60 mmHg. The perineum is intact, but heavy vaginal bleeding was observed.

19. A 28-year-old woman in her third pregnancy has an uneventful first- and second-stage labour. The placenta is delivered by continuous cord traction. Shortly after delivery of the placenta she complains of severe abdominal pain and collapses. On examination her pulse is 45 beats/minute and her blood pressure is 60/30 mmHg. On abdominal examination her uterus is not palpable.

Answers: MCQs

1. A False

    B True

    C True

    D False

    E True

    Pregnancy increases the incidence of cardiac arrhythmia. This is the result of hormonal changes, alterations in autonomic tone, increased haemodynamic demands and mild hypokalaemia. There is a 7% mortality rate with NYHA class III or IV and a risk of heart failure, irreversible left ventricular dysfunction and fetal loss.

2. A False

    B False

    C True

    D False

    E True

    Clinical disease activity follows the titre of thyroid-stimulating hormone receptor (TSH) receptor stimulating antibodies, which rises in the first trimester and puerperium and falls in the second and third trimesters. Carbimazole causes aplasia cutis congenita of the scalp in the infant, a rare congenital defect affecting 0.03% of the general population. More extensive and recent work indicates, however, that this association is either spurious or, at most, extremely rare and should not influence the choice of drug in pregnancy. TSH receptor stimulating antibodies cross the placenta and the risk of fetal Graves' disease after 20 weeks (the gestational age at which the fetal thyroid can respond to these antibodies) is directly proportional to their titre (although even at the highest titres, the risk is very low).

3. A False

    B True

    C True

    D False

    E True

    Chest infections should be managed aggressively. Hospital admission may be required for chest physiotherapy and administration of intravenous antibiotics. The Cystic Fibrosis Trust recommends performing an oral glucose tolerance test in the first trimester and at 24–28 weeks of gestation in all women who have normal glucose tolerance prior to pregnancy.

4. A False
    B True
    C True
    D False
    E False

    Data in the literature indicate that although tumour enlargement is only 3% for microprolactinomas, it is as high as 32% for macroprolactinomas that were not previously operated on. The current literature demonstrates that pregnancy induces remission of hyperprolactinaemia in two-thirds of women after discontinuation of dopamine antagonist. The patient should undergo baseline formal visual field testing at the time of diagnosis and should be followed clinically every 2–3 months during pregnancy, but serial MRI examinations or visual field testing during pregnancy is not required. However, there is no data documenting harm to the fetus from either MRI scans or gadolinium.

5. A False
    B False
    C False
    D True
    E False

    Based on recent evidence the National Institute for Health and Care Excellence (NICE) guidelines stipulate the need to give only 1 mg of parenteral vitamin K at birth to all children born to mothers taking enzyme-inducing anti-epileptic drugs (AEDs). Based on current evidence, routine monitoring of serum AED levels in pregnancy is not recommended. Enzyme-inducing AEDs such as phenytoin, carbamazepine and phenobarbitone may increase their metabolism of corticosteroids and reduce their therapeutic effectiveness. No study has assessed the effectiveness of higher or frequent doses of corticosteroids on neonatal outcomes in women at risk of preterm delivery and enzyme-inducing AEDs. Pethidine is metabolised to norpethidine which has been shown to be epileptogenic when administered in high doses to patients with normal renal function. It should therefore be avoided or used with caution.

6. A True
    B False
    C True
    D False
    E False

    A successful renal transplant restores fertility in young women. The glomerular filtration rate increases in normal pregnancy by 30–35% during the first two trimesters and decreases during the third trimester. If the functions of the transplanted kidneys are stable then it behaves like a normal kidney. The vast majority of women with a transplanted kidney are already hypertensive and are on medical treatment, even before pregnancy. Increased blood pressure occurs as a result of an increase in systematic vascular resistance. There is also an raised risk of pre-eclampsia. Cyclosporins should not be discontinued; in fact the dose requirement increases during pregnancy. Stopping immunosuppressive treatment can lead to acute rejection. Cyclosporins cross the placenta and increase the risk of intrauterine growth restriction. Most women on cyclosporins develop hypertension, hyperlipidaemia, nephrotoxicity, neurotoxicity and hepatotoxicity.

Answers: SBAs

7. A Women taking lithium should be changed immediately to an alternative upon becoming pregnant

Although lithium is teratogenic, some of the risks of fetal exposure may have been overplayed in the past, and abrupt cessation of treatment can lead to a relapse of the mood disorder. Furthermore, many women will only present for antenatal care after the most critical fetal developmental period. Nevertheless, alternatives are usually introduced in a controlled manner. Neonatal hypothyroidism and diabetes insipidus are recognised toxic side effects and breastfeeding is not recommended for women where lithium is reintroduced soon after delivery. This can be very important in helping to prevent a perinatal recurrence, the risk of which is as high as 50%. Both postpartum new-onset bipolar affective disorders and recurrences tend to present within the first week following delivery.

8. C Ibuprofen

Non-steroidal anti-inflammatory drugs, such as ibuprofen, are usually avoided in pregnancy because they have been associated with implantation failure and later on with fetal renal dysfunction and premature closure of the ductus arteriosus. Sumatriptan is a 5-hydroxytryptamine receptor antagonist, which has been used in pregnancy without obvious harmful effects. Data remains limited and the risk–benefit analysis should be carefully weighed-up in discussion with the woman. There is abundant experience with amitriptyline, and particularly with the low doses used in migraine prophylaxis no significant fetal concerns exist. Ergot alkaloids may cause placental vasoconstriction and should be avoided. Prophylaxis with the calcium-channel blocker verapamil is acceptable.

Answers: EMQs

9. B Peripartum cardiomyopathy

Peripartum cardiomyopathy (PPCM) is a form of dilated cardiomyopathy that is defined as deterioration in cardiac function presenting typically between the last month of pregnancy and up to 6 months postpartum. As with other forms of dilated cardiomyopathy, PPCM involves systolic dysfunction of the heart with a decrease of the left ventricular ejection fraction with associated congestive heart failure and an increased risk of atrial and ventricular arrhythmias, thromboembolism and even sudden cardiac death.

PPCM is a diagnosis of exclusion, wherein patients have no prior history of heart disease and there are no other known possible causes of heart failure. Echocardiogram is used to both diagnose and monitor the effectiveness of treatment for PPCM.

The cause of PPCM is unknown. Currently, researchers are investigating cardiotropic viruses, autoimmunity or immune system dysfunction, other toxins that serve as triggers to immune system dysfunction, micronutrient or trace mineral deficiencies, and genetics as possible components that contribute to or cause the development of PPCM.

10. K Pulmonary embolism

Pregnancy is a prothrombotic state. The incidence of thromboembolism is up to ten times higher in pregnant women than women of the same age who are not pregnant. Venous thromboembolism occurs throughout pregnancy, but the risk is about four-fold higher in the puerperium. The symptoms and signs of pulmonary embolism include sudden onset pleuritic chest pain, shortness of breath, haemoptysis, faintness or collapse, tachycardia, tachypnoea and raised jugular venous pressure.

Clinical assessment of VTE is not reliable for diagnosis. Only 5% of women with clinical signs of pulmonary embolism will have pulmonary thromboembolus (PTE) confirmed. Any woman with symptoms and signs suggestive of a PTE should have objective testing performed as soon as possible, and such women should be started on treatment with low molecular weight heparin (LMWH) until the diagnosis is excluded by objective testing.

11. B Thrombotic thrombocytopenic purpura

Thrombotic thrombocytopenic purpura (TTP) is a rare blood disorder characterised by clotting in small blood vessels of the body (thromboses), resulting in a low platelet count. In its full-blown form, the disease consists of the pentad of microangiopathic haemolytic anaemia, thrombocytopenic purpura, neurologic abnormalities, fever, and renal disease.

12. I Haemolytic uraemic syndrome

Haemolytic uremic syndrome (HUS) is primarily a disease of infancy and early childhood and is classically characterised by the triad of microangiopathic haemolytic anaemia, thrombocytopenia, and acute renal failure

13. H Disseminated intravascular coagulation

Disseminated intravascular coagulation (DIC) is characterised by systemic activation of blood coagulation, which results in generation and deposition of fibrin, leading to microvascular thrombi in various organs and contributing to multiple organ dysfunction syndrome. Consumption and subsequent exhaustion of coagulation proteins and platelets (from ongoing activation of coagulation) may induce severe bleeding, though micro-clot formation may occur in the absence of severe clotting factor depletion and bleeding.

14. D Acute fatty liver of pregnancy

Acute fatty liver of pregnancy (AFLP) is a serious complication unique to pregnancy first described by Sheehan in 1940. It is characterised by microvesicular steatosis in the liver. The foremost cause of AFLP is thought to be due to a mitochondrial dysfunction in the oxidation of fatty acids leading to an accumulation in hepatocytes. The infiltration of fatty acids causes acute liver insufficiency, which leads to most of the symptoms that present in this condition. If not diagnosed and treated promptly, AFLP can result in high maternal and neonatal morbidity and mortality.

The exact pathophysiology of AFLP is unknown. There does not appear to be a predilection for any geographical area or race. It appears to occur more commonly in primiparous women than multiparous women. Women who develop AFLP are more likely to have a heterozygous long-chain 3-hydroxyacyl-coenzyme A dehydrogenase (LCHAD) deficiency.

15. A HELLP syndrome

HELLP syndrome is a life-threatening liver disorder thought to be a variant of severe pre-eclampsia. It is characterised by haemolysis (destruction of red blood cells), elevated liver enzymes (which indicate liver damage) and low platelet count.

HELLP is usually related to pre-eclampsia. About 10–20% of women who have severe pre-eclampsia develop HELLP. In most cases, this happens before 35 weeks of pregnancy, though it can also develop right after childbirth.

16. I Cervical trauma

Cervical tears and trauma are a common cause of traumatic postpartum haemorrhage. Vaginal tears are common after rotational forceps delivery.

17. M Torsion of an ovarian cyst

Torsion of the ovarian cyst happens commonly after delivery due to laxity of the tissues.

18. F Atonic postpartum haemorrhage

Atonic postpartum haemorrhage is the most likely cause of the shock.

19. E Uterine inversion

Abdominal pain followed by collapse and a nonpalpable uterus suggests uterine inversion.

Chapter 5

Intrapartum care

Questions: SBAs

For each question, select the single best answer from the five options listed.

1. A woman is in labour under epidural for her first pregnancy at term. She has been fully dilated for 3 hours and pushed for an hour (the total duration of second stage was 3 hours). The vertex is still not visible. On abdominal examination 0/5th of the head is palpable and on pelvic examination the cervix is fully dilated with the vertex at the level of spine +1. The pelvis is adequate with no caput or moulding. The position is likely to be direct occipito-posterior.

    What is the best method of delivery in this circumstance?

    A Haig Ferguson forceps in the room
    B Ventouse delivery in the room
    C Manual rotation followed by Haig Ferguson forceps in theatre
    D Trial of rotational instrumental delivery in theatre
    E Caesarean section

2. A woman is in labour under epidural for her first pregnancy at term. She has been fully dilated for 2 hours and pushed for an hour. The vertex is not visible. She is contracting 2 per 10 minutes and her cardiotocography is normal. Abdominal and pelvic examinations show that 2/5th of the head is palpable. The cervix is fully dilated; the position is direct occipito-anterior with the vertex at the level of the spine. The pelvis is adequate with no large caput or moulding.

    What should the next step be?

    A Perform Haig Ferguson forceps in the room
    B Perform ventouse delivery in the room
    C Commence oxytocin
    D Trial instrumental delivery in theatre
    E Perform a caesarean section

Questions: EMQs

Question 3 – 6

Option list for questions 3 – 6:

A Intravenous adrenaline
B Caesarean section under spinal anaesthesia
C Chest X-ray and antibiotics
D Intramuscular adrenaline
E Category I caesarean section
F Wait and watch
G Caesarean section under gas induction

H Phenylephrine
I Epidural patch
J Opioid analgesia
K Subcutaneous adrenaline
L Check airway/breathing/circulation
M Fetal blood sampling
N Head-down position
O Caesarean section under epidural anaesthesia

For each case below, choose the single most appropriate action from the above list of options. Each option may be used once, more than once, or not at all.

3. A 32-year-old primigravid woman is being induced at 37 weeks' gestation for pre-eclampsia. Her blood pressure is 145/95 mmHg. She is asymptomatic. Her initial cardiotocography (CTG) is normal. She requests pain relief, and an epidural is sited. Her blood pressure falls suddenly to 85/55 mmHg. The CTG shows decelerations with spontaneous recovery. Intravenous fluids are given, and maternal hypotension is persistent with maternal tachycardia of 140 beats/minute.

4. A 34-year-old woman undergoes an elective lower-segment caesarean section (LSCS) for previous LSCS and maternal request. She has an uncomplicated procedure, but on the fifth postoperative day she complains of feeling unwell and being unable to care for her child due to severe headache. Simple analgesics are not helpful.

5. A 25-year-old primigravid woman is admitted in spontaneous labour at 40 weeks' gestation. She has a prolonged first stage, and fetal decelerations, for which she undergoes category II caesarean section under spinal anaesthesia. She is complaining of numbness at the level of her nipple and becomes breathless.

6. A 29-year-old primigravid woman presents in spontaneous labour at term. On vaginal examination a prolapsed pulsating cord is felt. She is rushed to theatre for a category 1 caesarean section. Her body mass index is 36, and there is difficulty in intubation.

Question 7 – 9

Option list for Questions 7 – 9:

A Fetal blood sample and forceps delivery in the delivery room
B Category I caesarean section
C Ventouse delivery in the delivery room

D Analgesia
E Fetal blood sampling and forceps delivery in theatre
F Forceps delivery in theatre

G   Fetal blood sampling and rotational forceps delivery in theatre
H   Category II caesarean section
I   Commence syntocinon infusion
J   Rotational forceps in the delivery room

K   Allow a further 30 minutes of active pushing
L   Rotational forceps in theatre
M   None of the above

For each case below, choose the single most appropriate management option from the above list of options. Each option may be used once, more than once, or not at all.

7. A 24-year-old woman at term is admitted in spontaneous labour and has progressed to full dilatation. She has been actively pushing for an hour. On abdominal examination the head is 0/5th palpable. Vaginal examination reveals the position is direct occipitoanterior, there is no caput and moulding, and the station is 2 cm below the ischial spines.

8. A 25-year-old primigravid woman at term is admitted in spontaneous labour. She progresses to full dilatation. She has been actively pushing for an hour. On abdominal examination the head is 0/5th palpable. On vaginal examination the midwife is unable to determine the position. The station is at the level of the ischial spines.

9. A 34-year-old woman at term is admitted in spontaneous labour and progresses to full dilatation. She has been actively pushing for an hour. On abdominal examination the head is 0/5th palpable. Vaginal examination reveals left occipitotransverse position, and there is evidence of moulding and caput. The station is 1 cm below the ischial spines.

Question 10 – 12

Option list for Questions 10 – 12:

A   Descent
B   Extension
C   Engagement
D   Flexion

E   External rotation
F   Restitution
G   Internal rotation
H   None of the above

For each description below, choose the single most appropriate mechanism from the above list of options. Each option may be used once, more than once, or not at all.

10. After the head delivers through the vulva, it immediately aligns with the fetal shoulders.

11. The occiput escapes from underneath the symphysis pubis, which acts as a fulcrum.

12. When the widest part of the presenting part has passed successfully through the pelvic inlet

Answers: SBAs

1. E Caesarean section

Knowing the position is one of the essential prerequisites before carrying instrumental delivery. If there is doubt about the position, assistance from a senior colleague should be sought. Since this option was not given. Then the safest thing to do is caesarean section.

2. C Commence oxytocin

Instrumental delivery is contraindicated if the head is >1/5th palpable per abdomen. The other two options are caesarean section and oxytocin. A caesarean is indicated if fetal distress or if there are signs of obstructed labour particularly in presence of adequate contractions. In this case contractions were not adequate and cardiotocography is normal. Therefore, the best answer will be to commence oxytocin.

Answers: EMQs

3. H Phenylephrine

Hypotension following epidural anaesthesia usually settles down with intravenous fluids. If it is persistent, the anaesthetist could consider sympathomimetics. Transient hypotension is well tolerated by an otherwise healthy fetus. Persistent fetal distress is an indication for immediate delivery.

4. I Epidural patch

Post-spinal headache occurs in 2% of cases following epidural anaesthesia and can be managed with a blood patch.

5. L Check airway/breathing/circulation

Spinal anaesthesia, can cause complications, some of them are life-threatening. Some of these complications are:

- Hypotension (spinal shock) due to sympathetic nervous system blockade. This is common and is usually easily treated with intravenous fluid and sympathomimetic drugs such as ephedrine, phenylephrine or metaraminol
- Postdural puncture headache (PDPH) or post-spinal headache, which is associated with the size and type of spinal needle used
- Cauda equina injury, although this very rare due to the insertion site being too high
- Cardiac arrest, although this is also very rare and usually related to the underlying medical condition of the patient

Because this is an acute emergency, management should start with the ABC. This is the basic principle in the management of any emergency situation.

6. G Caesarean section under gas induction

General anaesthesia is an option for category I caesarean sections. Obese pregnant women should ideally receive antenatal anaesthetic input.

7. C Chest X-ray and antibiotics

Instrumental delivery is indicated. The station is 2 cm below the spine. Delivery can be accomplished with the use of a ventouse cup in the delivery room.

8. F Forceps delivery in theatre

The likely reason for a delay in second stage is malposition of the fetal head. Examination in theatre and delivery by forceps after manual rotation or rotational forceps delivery is appropriate.

9. M None of the above

A confirmed transverse position of the fetal head with adequate descent into the pelvis may be managed by delivery with rotational forceps in theatre.

10. F Forceps delivery in theatre

Restitution is the passive movement of shoulders to align with the head after passage through the vulva.

11. B Extension

The process of delivery of the fetal head is completed by extension. The anterior shoulder lies inferior to the symphysis pubis and delivers first, and the posterior shoulder delivers subsequently.

12. C Engagement

Engagement is when the widest part of the fetal head passes through the inlet. The mechanism of labour refers to the series of changes that occur in the position and attitude of the fetus during its passage through the birth canal. The process involves engagement, descent, flexion, internal rotation, extension, restitution, external rotation and delivery of the shoulders and fetal body. Engagement is said to have occurred when the widest part of the presenting part has passed successfully through the pelvic inlet.

Chapter 6

Intrapartum care – complicated

Questions: MCQs

Answer each stem 'True' or 'False'.

1. **Successful trial of vaginal birth after caesarean section is influenced by:**
    A Epidural analgesia during labour
    B Attempted trial of vaginal birth at 39 weeks' gestation
    C Spontaneous onset of labour
    D Female infant
    E Estimated birth weight in current pregnancy

Questions: SBAs

For each question, select the single best answer from the five options listed.

2. Regarding face presentation:

    A The most favourable position for vaginal delivery is mentoanterior
    B It is associated with congenital anomalies
    C Continuous external fetal monitoring should be utilised
    D An instrumental delivery by ventouse or forceps can be performed in the event of prolonged second stage
    E An experienced neonatal practitioner should be present at the delivery

3. A 23-year-old woman in her first pregnancy is in labour at term. There was a delay in progress in the first stage of labour. The baby is of average size with no signs of obstruction. She is contracting 3–4 per 10 minutes. The next step should be:

    A Caesarean section for failure to progress
    B Commence augmentation with oxytocin
    C Continuous electronic fetal monitoring (or cardiotocography)
    D Perform abdominal and pelvic examination
    E Intravenous line, blood for group and save and attention must be made to ensure adequate hydration

4. You are called to labour ward to see a patient who has been admitted with regular contractions and intact membranes at 28 weeks' gestation. On speculum and vaginal examination, her cervix is 6 cm dilated and the presentation is cephalic.

    What is the most appropriate next course of action?

    A Consider a cervical suture
    B Administer atosiban to stop preterm labour
    C Administer the first dose of steroid for lung maturity
    D Administer erythromycin to prevent infection
    E Administer magnesium sulphate for fetal neuro-protection

5. Regarding umbilical cord prolapse, which of the following is not true?

    A Postmaturity
    B Prematurity
    C Grand multiparity
    D Kielland's rotational forceps delivery
    E Breech presentation

Answers: MCQs

1. A False

    B False

    C True

    D False

    E False

    Epidural anaesthesia does not decrease the likelihood of successful outcome. Outcome of a trial of vaginal birth is dependent on the cervical status in labour as a favourable cervical status increases the likelihood of a successful outcome independent of gestational age. It is believed that male infants decrease the likelihood of a successful outcome. The accuracy of ultrasound scan estimation of birth weight is operator-experience dependent and in itself is not a strong predictor of a successful outcome of labour.

Answers: SBAs

2. D An instrumental delivery by ventouse or forceps can be performed in the event of prolonged second stage

A fetus in a mentoposterior position cannot usually deliver vaginally unless the fetus is particularly preterm. This is because the fetal neck is already at maximum extension and cannot extend under the symphysis to allow for a vaginal delivery. If rotation to mentoanterior position occurs then vaginal delivery may be achievable; otherwise a caesarean section is indicated. Face presentation is associated with congenital anomalies that are associated with neck extension such as neck masses, or where the size of the head is not fitting into the pelvis normally such as ventriculomegaly. Continuous external fetal monitoring should be utilised in all cases when face presentation has been diagnosed, as there is an increased risk of a lower cord pH at delivery and lower Apgar scores. An instrumental delivery by forceps can be considered in face presentation, but a ventouse must not be used as it could cause damage to the facial structures especially the eyes. An experienced neonatal practitioner should be present at delivery since there is an increased risk of lower Apgar scores and a risk of neck oedema necessitating intubation.

3. C Continuous electronic fetal monitoring (or cardiotocography)

For failure to progress either in first or second stage the first priority is to ensure fetal well-being by continuous cardiotocography (CTG) monitoring. Next priority is to establish IV access, hydration and to send blood for group and save. One of the features associated with poor uterine activity is dehydration. It is therefore important to ensure adequate hydration for women with delay in the first stage of labour. An abdominal and pelvic examination should then be performed. If there are signs of fetal compromise or signs of obstructed labour like moulding, caput or haematuria especially in presence of adequate uterine activity, then CS is indicated. Otherwise augmentation with oxytocin will be needed. In this case the answer will be continuous CTG monitoring.

4. C Administer the first dose of steroid for lung maturity

A cervical suture is of no benefit at this gestation. Although Atosiban may delay delivery for up to 7 days, but it has no role when labour is advanced. Routine use of antibiotics in the presence of intact membranes is not of benefit without clinical evidence of infection, and in fact the ORACLE II study suggested that they may be associated with harm. Magnesium sulphate is of no use as a tocolytic, but some evidence supports its use for fetal nuroprotection. A steroid for lung maturity has the best evidence of all other interventions even if delivery is imminent and it should always be considered first.

5. A Postmaturity

Umbilical cord prolapse is more common when the presenting part does not fit well in the maternal pelvis. This includes prematurity, grand multiparity and breech presentation.

In Kielland's forceps delivery the head may need disimpaction from the pelvis before rotation can be affected, hence the increased chance of cord prolapse.

Chapter 7

Obstetric operations and emergency interventions

Questions: MCQs

Answer each stem 'True' or 'False'.

1. **Regarding placenta praevia:**
    - A   Transvaginal ultrasound scan should not be used for the diagnosis of placenta praevia in the third trimester
    - B   MRI scan at 36 weeks is 95% sensitive to rule out placenta accreta
    - C   Elective caesarean section should be planned for all women with major placenta praevia at 36 weeks' gestation
    - D   Women with major placenta praevia should not be offered home-based care
    - E   When a low lying placenta is noted at routine mid trimester scan, then a confirmatory scan should be carried out at 32 weeks

2. **When management of morbidly adherent placenta:**
    - A   MRI scanning has 100% sensitivity in making an accurate diagnosis of placenta accreta
    - B   Gray's scale ultrasound scan with colour Doppler flow has a sensitivity up to 100%
    - C   Regional anaesthesia should not be used for delivery of women with placenta praevia
    - D   The prophylactic placement of arterial catheters prior to elective caesarean section reduces risk of major postpartum haemorrhage
    - E   Conservative management of a retained placenta following delivery with adjuvant methotrexate treatment is effective

3. **The following risk factors have been linked to placenta praevia**
    - A   Advanced maternal age (>40 years)
    - B   Deficient endometrium due to the presence of submucous fibroid
    - C   Multiple pregnancy
    - D   Previous placenta praevia
    - E   Previous termination of pregnancy

Questions: SBAs

For each question, select the single best answer from the five options listed.

4. Regarding external cephalic version, which is the following is correct?

    A It is successful in approximately half of all attempts
    B It is completely contraindicated with a history of previous caesarean section
    C It must not be attempted in labour
    D It is less likely to be successful if tocolysis is used
    E It should not be performed after 40 weeks' gestation

5. An antenatal screening test for gestational diabetes mellitus (GDM) was evaluated in 100 primigravid women, and 20 of them were screen-positive. At the end of the study only 10 women developed GDM; only 5 of these were among the twenty screen-positive women.

   Which of the following statements is correct?

    A Sensitivity of the test is 25%
    B Specificity of the test is 10%
    C Positive predictive value of the test is 50%
    D Negative predictive value of the test is 5%
    E Test would be expected to have similar performance if applied to the whole pregnant population (primigravid and multigravid)

	+	-	
+	10(a)	10(b)	20
-	5(c)	75(d)	80

6. Regarding principles within medical negligence law:

    A In a medical negligence claim, the standard of proof required is 'on a balance of probabilities'
    B The Bolam defence preceded the Bolitho case
    C It is enough to defend a doctor if a body of experts support his/her actions
    D Proving 'breach of duty' is sufficient for a successful medical negligence claim
    E There is no difference between an expert and a professional witness

7. Which of the following cannot be attributed to 'latent' causes of clinical risk?

    A Poor staffing levels
    B Unprofessional behaviour
    C Inadequate training
    D Absence of clinical guidelines
    E Lack of supervision

8. Regarding methods of termination of pregnancy:

    A   Surgical methods have marginally higher success rates than medical
    B   Mifepristone and misoprostol are not licensed for medical termination at 8 weeks' gestation
    C   Mifepristone is not teratogenic
    D   The delay between mifepristone and misoprostol administration can be reduced to less than 24 hours without affecting success rates
    E   Gemeprost can be used as an alternative to mifepristone.

Questions: EMQs

Question 9 – 11

Option list for Questions 9 – 11:

A   Inform the anaesthetist and senior surgeon, and perform an end-to-end anastomosis

B   Interrupted non-absorbable sutures and a catheter in situ for 10 days

C   Caesarean hysterectomy

D   Inform the anaesthetist and senior surgeon, and perform two-layer closure of the small bowel with absorbable sutures

E   Single-layer closure

F   Two-layer closure with absorbable sutures, with a catheter in situ for 2 days

G   B Lynch suture

H   Defunctioning colostomy

I   Right haemicolectomy

J   Intramyometrial carboprost

K   Two-layer closure with nonabsorbable sutures and a catheter in situ for 2 days

L   Interventional radiology and bilateral uterine artery embolisation

M   Expectant management

N   Interrupted absorbable sutures and a catheter in situ for 10 days

O   Unilateral ligation of the uterine artery

P   Inform the anaesthetist and senior surgeon, and perform two-layer closure of the small bowel with nonabsorbable sutures

Q   Bilateral ligation of the uterine arteries

For each description below, choose the single most appropriate answer from the above list of options. Each option may be used once, more than once, or not at all.

9.   A 28-year-old woman who is para 1, with a previous caesarean section, undergoes an elective repeat caesarean section. Difficulties are encountered during entry into the peritoneal cavity. The patient's urine is blood-stained at the end of surgery. A methylene blue test shows a 2 cm defect in the dome of the bladder.

10. A 32-year-old woman undergoes elective surgery for a breech presentation at 38 weeks' gestation. She is known to have undergone bowel surgery as a child. Difficulty is encountered during entry into the peritoneal cavity. After delivery of the fetus, faecal soiling is noted in the peritoneal cavity. Further exploration reveals a 1 cm size defect in the small bowel.

11. A 29-year-old woman who is a Jehovah's Witness undergoes a repeat caesarean section for a placenta praevia. Massive postpartum haemorrhage is encountered. The initial medical management and placement of a B-Lynch suture are unsuccessful.

Answers: MCQs

1. A False

    B False

    C False

    D False

    E False

    Transvaginal ultrasound scan is not contraindicated in the diagnosis of placenta praevia. It is superior to transabdominal ultrasonography in the diagnosis of posterior placenta praevia. When a low-lying placenta is suspected during second trimester scanning, a repeat image should be performed around 32 weeks' gestation to clarify the diagnosis. Home-based care is not contraindicated for women with major placenta praevia provided they live in close proximity to the hospital of confinement and there is no issue regarding their transport. Elective caesarean delivery for asymptomatic women is not recommended before 38 weeks of gestation for placenta praevia. MRI scan does not have a very high sensitivity, therefore it cannot rule out placenta accreta.

2. A False

    B True

    C False

    D False

    E False

    The role of MRI scan remains unclear whereas Gray's scale ultrasound scan complemented by colour Doppler and 3D Doppler remains the imaging modality of choice with sensitivity up to 100% and specificity up to 85%. The value of prophylactic placement of arterial catheters at the time of delivery for suspected cases of placenta accreta remains unclear. Regional anaesthesia is not contraindicated for delivery of placenta praevia and this decision should be made in consultation with other members of the multidisciplinary team. The use of methotrexate in this situation remains unclear as there will be no ongoing active mitotic activity. It is highly unlikely that methotrexate use will facilitate resolution of this condition and reduce the risk of bleeding. Close monitoring of such patients is mandated to manage the risk of haemorrhage.

3. A True

    B True

    C True

    D True

    E True

A number of risk factors for placenta praaevia have been described. These risk factors are often related to conditions that existed prior to pregnancy. Multiparity, previous caesarean section, deficient endometrium (secondary to uterine scar, endometritis, curettage, sub mucous fibroid, vigorous curettage) multiple pregnancies, smoking and advanced maternal age are well recognised risk factors.

Answers: SBAs

4. A It is successful in approximately half of all attempts

External cephalic version (ECV) is successful in only 50% of cases in many series from the UK, although this success rate is higher for multiparous women and also when tocolysis is used routinely. Early labour with intact membranes and previous caesarean section are not absolute contraindications to ECV, nor is a gestation beyond 40 weeks.

5. C Positive predictive value of the test is 50%

Sensitivity (=a/a+c) is the probability that the test will be positive if the condition is present.

Specificity (=d/b+d) is the probability that the test will be negative if the condition is absent. Positive predictive value (=a/a+b) is the probability that the condition is present if the test is positive. Negative predictive value (=d/c+d) is the probability that the condition is absent if the test is negative. The test will not have the same performance in the whole population because the prevalance of condition (GDM) is different between the study population (primigravid) and the whole population (primigravid and multigravid).

6. C It is enough to defend a doctor if a body of experts support his/her actions

In a civil negligence claim (e.g. medical negligence) the standard of proof required is 'on a balance of probabilities' (i.e. more than 50% likely). Criminal claims require 'beyond all reasonable doubt'. The Bolitho case came after the Bolam defence and effectively meant that it was no longer sufficient for a group of doctors to support the actions of an accused doctor if a claim was to be effectively defended. The Bolitho case modified this so that the court also had to be satisfied that this opinion had a logical basis.

A successful medical negligence claim requires the claimant to show that there was a duty of care, that this was breached by the doctor, and lastly that this breach of duty caused, or contributed to, the damage (causation). Expert witnesses should give their opinions independent of whether they are instructed by a claimant or a defendant. It is not their job to argue the case on behalf of one party, or the other. A doctor may be asked to only give factual evidence, for example when explaining clinical notes, in particular the intervention or treatment received by the patient. They will therefore be a professional witness, not an expert witness.

An expert witness is also a professional witness but provides an expert opinion on the subject matter. Their duty is to assist the judge and jury with necessary scientific criteria to test their conclusions, so the judge or jury can form their own judgement. The scientific evidence provided by the expert is an important factor for consideration by the court, but along with other evidence it is the judge or jury who makes final decision.

7. B Unprofessional behaviour

Latent causes of risk are those causes inherent to the department or hospital which increase the chance that a clinician will make an error. They are 'remote' from the actual incident. Poor staffing levels, inadequate training/supervision and an absence of clinical guidelines are all examples. Failure to adhere to guidelines and poor attitudes are risk issues relevant to individuals and are often the immediate cause of a patient safety incident.

8. D The delay between mifepristone and misoprostol administration can be reduced to less than 24 hours without affecting success rates

All accepted methods of termination of pregnancy have high rates of success (95% and above), however surgical success rates are marginally better (98–99%) than medical (95–98%). Although mifepristone and misoprostol are used in combination at all gestations from 4 weeks for medical termination, they are only licensed up to 49 days. Between 9 and 13 weeks, the failure rate is slightly higher, as are rates of significant haemorrhage. There is no evidence that mifepristone is teratogenic; this belief is important for that small group of women who change their minds about medical termination after taking the mifepristone and before the misoprostol. Misoprostol may be less benign, and anomalies have been reported in pregnancies which have continued following failed misoprostol treatment. Traditionally 48 hours was left between the ingestion of mifepristone and the administration of misoprostol, however there is evidence that this can be reduced to 24 hours. However, leaving even less time than this does seem to increase failure rates. Gemeprost is licensed for use in medical termination, and is used following prior ingestion of mifepristone.

9. N Interrupted absorbable sutures and a catheter in situ for 10 days

The incidence of bladder damage during caesarean section is about 0.3%. The bladder wall can be repaired by a single continuous or interrupted technique. Postoperatively, the catheter needs to be in situ for at least a week.

10. D Inform the anaesthetist and senior surgeon, and perform two-layer closure of the small bowel with absorbable sutures

Bowel damage is extremely rare during caesarean section and needs full exploration.

Small bowel can be repaired in two layers, but large bowel damage requires a temporary defunctioning colostomy.

11. C Caesarean hysterectomy

In cases of repeat caesarean section with placenta praevia, postpartum haemorrhage should be anticipated and early hysterectomy could be life-saving. Up to 30% of caesarean hysterectomies are done for this indication.

Chapter 8

Postnatal care

Questions: MCQs

Answer each stem 'True' or 'False'.

1. **Regarding postpartum haemorrhage:**
    - A An estimated blood loss of 1.5 litres for an average woman weighing 70 kg is life-threatening
    - B Prophylactic oxytocics in the management of third stage of labour reduces the risk of postpartum haemorrhage by 90%
    - C During caesarean section 10 IU of oxytocin should be administered rapidly following delivery of the baby
    - D Ergometrine should not be used as prophylaxis
    - E Misoprostol is as effective as oxytocin for the prevention of postpartum haemorrhage

2. **Risk factors for postpartum haemorrhage:**
    - A Delayed cord clamping increases risk for postpartum haemorrhage
    - B Pre-gestational hypertension increases risk of PPH
    - C Gestational diabetes mellitus (GDM)/type 2 DM increases risk of PPH
    - D Active management of third stage is associated with secondary postpartum haemorrhage
    - E Teenage pregnancy is a risk factor for postpartum haemorrhage (PPH)

Questions: SBAs

For each question, select the single best answer from the five options listed.

3. Which of the following statement best describes perinatal mortality?

    A   The number of stillbirths is included in the enumerator
    B   The total number of babies dying in the neonatal period is included in the
        enumerator
    C   The total number of live birth is used as a denominator
    D   Babies dying as a result of lethal congenital abnormality are excluded
    E   Babies born dead before 28 weeks' gestation are not included

4. From the list of following drugs which one should be avoided during breastfeeding:

    A   Heparin
    B   Warfarin
    C   Ondansetron
    D   Metronidazole
    E   Phenindione

5. Regarding maternal mortality, which of the following is incorrect?

    A   It includes deaths up to 42 days after the termination of pregnancy
    B   Direct deaths are those resulting from obstetric complications of the pregnant
        state
    C   Includes fortuitous deaths
    D   Cardiac diseases are the most common cause of indirect death
    E   It includes direct and indirect deaths

Questions: EMQs

Question 6 – 8

Option list for Questions 6 – 8

A   All four position
B   Anticipate postpartum haemorrhage (PPH)
C   Check for perineal tears after delivery
D   Delivery of the posterior shoulder should be attempted
E   Episiotomy
F   Fundal pressure
G   Help should be summoned immediately
H   Internal rotation manoeuvre
I   Maternal pushing should be encouraged
J   McRobert's manoeuvre
K   Suction of baby's nostrils to avoid meconium aspiration
L   Suprapubic pressure
M   Watchful expectancy

For each case described below, choose the single most appropriate course of action from the list of options. Each option may be used once, more than once or not at all.

6.   A primigravid woman has been in the 2nd stage of labour for 2.5 hours. The head has been delivered by Haig Ferguson forceps. The liquor is meconium-stained, and there is difficulty in delivering the shoulders.

7.   A midwife is attending a home delivery of a 28-year-old woman in her second pregnancy at 39 weeks with body mass index of 22. The head remains tightly applied to the vulva and does not restitute.

8.   A registrar is attending a delivery of a 29-year-old woman in her second uneventful pregnancy at 39 weeks. Her previous pregnancy ended with a vaginal delivery complicated by a shoulder dystocia. The baby had a transient Erb's palsy. She is now fully dilated and the head is at the direct occipitoanterior position with no caput or moulding. She has been pushing for 20 minutes. The cardiotocography is normal.

Questions 9 – 11

Option list for Questions 9 – 11

A   Baby blues
B   Postnatal depression
C   Panic disorders
D   Schizophrenia
E   Puerperal psychosis
F   Bipolar affective disorder
G   Depression
H   Withdrawal psychosis
I   Personality disorder
J   Space-occupying lesions
K   Acute confusional state
L   Metabolic disorder
M   Post-traumatic stress disorder
N   None of the above

For each case below, choose the single most appropriate diagnosis from the above list of options. Each option may be used once, more than once, or not at all.

9. A 27-year-old woman who has had a normal delivery 10 hours earlier is noted by the ward staff to be having difficulties sleeping, is overactive and expresses feelings of excitement.

10. An 18-year-old woman presents at the booking clinic. She is 9 weeks into in her first pregnancy and has been referred by the community midwife for consultant care. She feels well in herself and says that a specific voice has been speaking to her every morning instructing her to do things. She is not on any medication.

11. A 36-year-old woman presents on the 4th day after a normal delivery. Her husband brought her in to the emergency department after he noticed an abrupt change in her behaviour. He describes her as confused, restless and expressing thoughts of self-harm.

Answers: MCQs

1. **A** False

   B False

   C False

   D False

   E False

   Because of the physiological expansion of blood volume at term, total blood volume will be around 7000 mL in these women. A blood loss of > 40% of total blood volume (approximately 2800 mL) will be generally regarded as life threatening. Prophylactic oxytocics reduce risk of primary postpartum haemorrhage (PPH) by about 60%. At caesarean section the common practice is to administer 5 IU of oxytocin by slow injection. Ergometrine is only contraindicated for prophylaxis on those women who are hypertensive. Ergometrine can still be used in life-threatening conditions when uterus is failing to contract. All evidence suggests that misoprostol, although effective in prevention ofPPH, is not as effective as oxytocin.

2. **A** False

   B True

   C False

   D False

   E False

   Delayed cord clamping has not been demonstrated to be associated with increased risk of PPH. Pre-eclampsia and gestational hypertension are known risk factors but gestational diabetes mellitus (GDM) is not. GDM-related increased risk of PPH may be related to size of the large baby or prolonged labour but itself is not a risk factor. Active management of the third stage does not increase the risk of secondary PPH. Risk of PPH is increased in elderly mothers, especially those over 40. Risk of PPH is higher among women of Asian ethnicity (odds ratio of 2).

Answers: SBAs

3. A The number of stillbirths is included in the enumerator

In calculating the perinatal mortality (PNM) rate, the enumerator includes the number of stillborn babies (i.e. those born with no signs of life at or after 24 completed weeks of gestation) and early perinatal deaths (babies dying during the first week of life, regardless of the gestational age at delivery), and the denominator is per 1000 total births. The neonatal period (first 4 weeks of life) is divided into early (first week) and late (the subsequent 3 weeks). PNM rates are the cornerstone for measuring obstetric care and are seen in the Western world as a measure of the quality of obstetric practice. Congenital malformations are one of the main causes of PNM, and sometimes what is called the 'corrected' PNM rate is calculated by excluding babies with lethal congenital anomalies.

4. E Phenindione

Phenindione is a synthetic anticoagulant which acts by interfering with the formation of factors II, VII, IX and X. Infants should not be fed with breast milk from mothers being treated with it. All the other medications are safe.

5. C Includes fortuitous deaths

Maternal mortality includes death of a woman while pregnant or within 42 days of pregnancy, irrespective of the duration and the site of the pregnancy, from any cause related to or aggravated by the pregnancy or its management but not from accidental or incidental causes (fortuitous). Direct deaths are those resulting from obstetric complications of the pregnant state (pregnancy, labour and the puerperium), from interventions, omissions, incorrect treatment, or from a chain of events resulting from any of the above.

Indirect deaths are those resulting from a previous existing disease or disease that developed during pregnancy, i.e. not due to direct causes, but which were aggravated by physiologic effects of pregnancy.

Answers: EMQs

6. G Help should be summoned immediately

Shoulder dystocia is a potentially life-threatening emergency requiring a team approach. Any individual obstetrician (or midwife) however skilled is more likely to succeed in dealing with shoulder dystocia if they have expert help. Therefore, summoning immediate help is the first step in management. The HELPERR mnemonic (from American Life Support Organization) has been devised to aid in remembering what to do in case of shoulder dystocia:

- H – Call for help
- E – Evaluate for episiotomy
- L – Legs (the McRoberts' manoeuvre)
- P – Suprapubic pressure
- E – Enter manoeuvres (internal rotation)
- R – Remove the posterior arm
- R – Roll the patient

7. A All fours position

All fours position is more appropriate when dealing with shoulder dystocia at community setting where immediate help is not available to do other manoeuvre like McRoberts'. The McRoberts' manoeuvre is more appropriate to be performed in hospital especially with women who have a high body mass index or are labouring under epidural.

8. M Watchful expectancy

There is no indication for intervention at this stage. Poor progress in second stage is defined as follows:

Nulliparous women – lack of continuing progress for 3 hours (total of active and passive second-stage labour) with regional anaesthesia, or 2 hours without regional anaesthesia.

Multiparous women – lack of continuing progress for 2 hours (total of active and passive second-stage labour) with regional anaesthesia, or 1 hour without regional anaesthesia.

The rate of shoulder dystocia in women who have had a previous shoulder dystocia has been reported to be 10 times higher than the rate in the general population. There is a reported recurrence rate of shoulder dystocia of between 1% and 25%. All birth attendants should be aware of the methods for diagnosing shoulder dystocia and the techniques required to facilitate delivery. There is no evidence that the use of the McRoberts' manoeuvre before delivery of the fetal head prevents shoulder dystocia. Therefore, prophylactic McRoberts' positioning before delivery of the fetal head is not recommended to prevent shoulder dystocia.

9. M Post-traumatic stress disorder

Many symptoms in the postnatal period may mimic psychiatric disorders, and a detailed history and careful evaluation are necessary.

10. D Schizophrenia

Auditory hallucinations, thought withdrawal, insertion and interruption, thought broadcasting, delusional perception and feelings or actions experienced as made or influenced by external agents are considered as first-rank symptoms of schizophrenia.

11. G Depression

The prevalence of postnatal depression is about 10%, but severe depression with suicidal thoughts is relatively less common. Immediate psychiatric evaluation, preferably in a mother and baby unit, is necessary.

Chapter 9

The newborn

Questions: MCQs

Answer each stem 'True' or 'False'.

1. **Regarding neonatal infection:**
    - A   Contact with birthing animals is associated with *Chlamydia psittaci* infection
    - B   Contact with aborting sheep is associated with Q fever (*Coxilla burnetti*) infection
    - C   Ingestion of milk products is associated with *Listeria* infection
    - D   The baby is especially at risk if the mother is infected with *Streptococcus* and *Staphylococcus* organisms.
    - E   Treat the baby with antibiotics only if the baby is infected with group A *Streptococcus*

2. **Regarding human immunodeficiency virus (HIV) transmission during pregnancy:**
    - A   All infants born to HIV-positive mothers have serum HIV antibodies
    - B   Serum HIV antibodies in infants are indicative of placental transmission
    - C   A positive HIV DNA PCR before 7 days indicates intrapartum transmission
    - D   HIV antibodies persist up to 18 months of age in infant serum
    - E   Duration of ruptured membranes has been associated with intrapartum transmission in women on effective highly active antiretroviral therapy (HAART) with undetectable viral loads

Questions: SBAs

For each question, select the single most appropriate answer from the five options listed.

3. A 26-year-old multiparous woman is in labour at term; there is thick meconium. She progressed well and had spontaneous vaginal delivery.

   Regarding resuscitation of her baby, which of the following is the most appropriate action to do?

   A   Nasopharyngeal suction should be performed with the head on the perineum, before the body has delivered
   B   Nasopharyngeal suction should be performed after delivery
   C   The newborn should be electively intubated at birth
   D   The newborn head should be kept in an extended position
   E   The mouth should be gently suctioned. Deep suctioning should only be done if there are signs of airway obstruction

4. A term newborn developed neonatal jaundice that appeared on the second day and is still present at 2 weeks of age.

   What is the most likely diagnosis from the following options?

   A   Haemolytic disease of the newborn due to rhesus incompatibility
   B   Galactosaemia
   C   Duodenal atresia
   D   Phenylketonuria
   E   Neonatal hyperthyroidism

Questions: EMQs

Question 5 – 9

Options list for Questions 5 – 9

A	Sensitivity	G	Likelihood ratio
B	Positive predictive value	H	True positive rate
C	Odds ratio	I	Negative predictive value
D	Screen positive rate	J	False positive rate
E	False negative rate	K	Specificity
F	Accuracy		

For each clinical scenario described below, choose the single most appropriate test from the list of options above. Each option may be used once, more than once or not at all.

5. The ability of a screening test to identify unaffected individuals

6. The likelihood that an individual screened positive for the condition actually has the disease

7. The proportion of individuals screened positive who do not actually have the condition

8. The proportion of the screened population who have a positive result

9. The ability of a test to identify affected individuals

Answers: MCQs

1. A False

   B False

   C True

   D True

   E False

   Antibiotic treatment is required if infection is noted in the mother, baby or both.

2. A True

   B False

   C False

   D True

   E False

   All infants born to HIV-positive mothers have serum HIV antibodies because of passive placental transfer, which persist up to 18 months of age; this does not indicate infection with the virus. A positive HIV DNA on PCR testing from the infant before 7 days of age indicates in utero transmission; if positive at 1 month this indicates intrapartum transmission, although the cut-offs are not absolute. Duration of ruptured membranes has been associated with intrapartum transmission in previous research, although new UK data show that this may not be the case for women on effective highly active antiretroviral therapy (HAART) with undetectable viral loads.

Answers: SBAs

3. E The mouth should be gently suctioned. Deep suctioning should only be done if there are signs of airway obstruction

Routine nasopharyngeal suction at any point, or intubation, is not recommended. Nasopharyngeal suctioning may induce a bradycardia. These manoeuvers should be reserved for babies with signs of upper airway obstruction, or those that fail to respond to initial resuscitative measures, including positive pressure ventilation by mask.

When resuscitating a newborn, care needs to be taken in maintaining a 'neutral' position. Flexion or extension at the neck can lead to obstruction of the airway.

4. B Galactosaemia

The main causes are inborn errors of metabolism, hepatic disorders and hypothyroidism.

Answers: EMQs

5. K Specificity

6. B Positive predictive value

7. J False positive rate

8. D The screen positive rate (false positives plus true positives)

9. A Sensitivity

Sensitivity is the ability of a test to correctly identify those with the disease (true positive rate), whereas specificity is the ability of the test to correctly identify those without the disease (true negative rate). Positive predictive value is the probability that subjects with a positive screening test truly have the disease. Negative predictive value is the probability that subjects with a negative screening test truly don't have the disease.

Section B

Gynaecology

Chapter 10

Basic reproductive endocrinology

Questions: MCQs

Answer each stem 'True' or 'False'.

1. **Raised prolactin:**
   - A   Is associated with polycystic ovarian syndrome
   - B   Can present with headaches and galactorrhoea
   - C   Is caused by risperidone
   - D   Causes menorrhagia
   - E   Causes dysmenorrhea

2. **Regarding oestrogen:**
   - A   Oestrone is the most potent oestrogen
   - B   Oestrone is the placental oestrogen
   - C   Oestriol is the least potent oestrogen
   - D   Oestradiol is the dominant oestrogen in the premenopause
   - E   Most oestradiol in the premenopause is produced by the aromatisation of androestenedione in peripheral (fatty) tissue

3. **Steroid hormones:**
   - A   Activate gene expression
   - B   Effects are seen within minutes   *Hour to days*
   - C   Cholesterol is the precursor to all steroid hormones
   - D   Progesterone is an example
   - E   Testosterone is an example

4. **In the follicular phase of menstrual cycle:**
   - A   Plasma oestrogen levels are low at the beginning
   - B   There is proliferation of the endometrial lining
   - C   Follicle-stimulating hormone rises initially
   - D   Luteinising hormone remains low until 1–2 days preovulation
   - E   Follicle-stimulating hormone is at its peak at the beginning of the follicular phase

5. **Dehydroepiandrosterone (DHEA):**
   - A   Is produced in the skin
   - B   Is an intermediate in the synthesis of androgen

  ✗ **C** Is a strong androgen
  ✓**D** Is usually found in the sulphate form in the blood
  ✗**E** Is absent in people with congenital androgen insensitivity syndrome

6. **Progesterone:**
  A Is a type of progestogen
  ✗**B** Is synthesised from deoxycorticosterone
  ✗**C** Is synthesised from androstenedione
  ✗**D** Is highest in the follicular phase of the menstrual cycle
  ✓**E** Is produced by the placenta

7. **Concerning steroidogenesis:**
  ✗**A** Aromatase converts dihydrotestosterone to oestradiol
  ✗**B** 5α-reductase converts testosterone to oestradiol
  C 17α-hydroxylase converts pregnenolone to 17α-hydroxypregnenolone
  ✓**D** 21 hydroxylase converts progesterone and 17α-hydroxyl progesterone to deoxycorticosterone and 11-deoxycortisol
  ✗**E** Cortisol is the precursor for 11-deoxycortisol

8. **Concerning testosterone:**
  A >90% is protein bound
  B Dihydrotestosterone is the most potent form
  ✓**C** Testosterone is converted to dihydrotestosterone by 5α-reductase
  D Most testosterone is bound to albumin *protein*
  ✗**E** Dihydrotesterone is five times less potent than testosterone

9. **Human chorionic gonadotropin:**
  A Has a subunit similar molecular structure to luteinising hormone, follicle-stimulating hormone and thyroid-stimulating hormone
  B Is a steroid *gluco prot*
  C Is composed of 337 amino acids   *237*
  D Promotes the maintenance of the corpus luteum during the beginning of the pregnancy
  ✓**E** Is produced by choriocarcinoma

10. **Hypogonadotrophic hypogonadism:**
  A The dysfunction is at the level of the hypothalamus and pituitary
  ✓**B** Is associated with low follicle-stimulating hormone
  C Can be caused by premature ovarian failure
  ✓**D** Is associated with low oestrogen
  E Can be caused by polycystic ovarian syndrome

11. **The following drugs may be associated with hyperprolactinaemia:**
  ✓**A** Methyldopa
  B Nifedipine
  C Fluoxetine
  ✓**D** Cocaine
  ✓**E** Danazol

Answers: MCQs

1. A True

    B True

    C True

    D False

    E False

    Prolactin is a 23 kDa polypeptide hormone secreted by the lactotroph cells of the anterior pituitary gland. It can be due to a prolactin producing tumour in the pituitary and therefore can present with headaches and visual disturbance.

    Raised prolactin typically causes oligomenorrhoea or secondary amenorrhoea. It is also mildly raised in polycystic ovarian syndrome.

    Drugs causing raised prolactin include: antipsychotics such as haloperidol and risperidone, antidepressants (tricyclic antidepressants such as amitriptyline, selective serotonin receptor re-uptake inhibitors such as sertraline, and monoamino oxidase inhibitors such as pargyline), prokinetics (e.g. metoclopramide), antihypertensive (e.g. methyldopa), H2 antagonists (e.g. cimetidine).

2. A False

    B False

    C True

    D True

    E False

    There are 3 types of oestrogen: oestrone (E1), oestradiol (E2), oestriol (E3). Oestrone is the oestrogen of the menopause. It is less potent than oestradiol and is produced by the aromatisation of androestenedione in peripheral (fatty) tissue, the adrenal gland and ovarian stroma. Oestradiol is the most potent oestrogen with the highest effect on oestrogen receptors. It is produced by the aromatisation of testosterone in the graafian follicle (granulosa cell). Oestriol is the placental oestrogen and is the least potent of all the oestrogens.

3. A True

    B False

    C True

    D True

    E True

    Steroid hormones diffuse across the plasma membrane and form complexes with cytosolic or nuclear receptors. After which the bound complex activates transcription of certain genes. Therefore, it takes hours to days for effects to manifest. Examples of steroid hormones include testosterone, oestrogen, progesterone and cortisol.

4. A True

   B True

   C True

   D True

   E False

The corpus luteum, which is the principal source of oestrogen during the luteal phase, has involutes before the follicular phase so oestrogen levels are low. Thus negative feedback is reduced and follicle-stimulating hormone (FSH) secretions begin to rise. This stimulates the development of several follicles, of which one will become the dominant follicle. The growing follicles secrete oestrogen that will inhibit FSH production in the latter part of the follicular phase. However, the dominant follicle becomes increasingly sensitive to circulating FSH and oestrogen continues to rise. When plasma oestrogen reaches a critical level it switches from negative feedback to positive feedback and stimulates a surge of FSH and luteinising hormone which cause rupture of the follicle and release of the egg.

5. A False

   B True

   C False

   D True

   E False

Dehydroepiandrosterone (DHEA) is an endogenous steroid hormone produced in the adrenal glands, gonads and brain. It is a weak androgen. It is usually found in the sulphate ester form in the blood (300 times more than free form).

6. A True

   B False

   C False

   D False

   E True

Progesterone is the main type of progestogen. It is synthesised from pregnenolone, which in turn is derived from cholesterol. It is found in low levels in the follicular phase of the menstrual cycle but levels rise in the luteal phase as it is produced by the corpus luteum. If pregnancy occurs the placenta begins to produce progesterone from approximately 7 weeks.

7. **A** False

   B False

   C True

   D True

   E False

   Aromatase converts androstenedione and testosterone to oestrone and oestradiol. 5α-reductase converts testosterone to dihydrotestosterone. 21 hydroxylase converts progesterone and 17α-hydroxyl progesterone to deoxycorticosterone and 11-deoxycortisol. 11-deoxycortisol is the precursor to cortisol converted by 11β-hydroxylase.

8. **A** True

   B True

   C True

   D False

   E False

   Testosterone is a steroid hormone. In women, it is synthesised by the thecal cells of the ovaries, the placenta, the zona reticularis of the adrenal cortex and even skin. Over 98% is bound to protein in plasma, most commonly sex hormone binding globulin and less commonly albumin. A small amount is converted to oestradiol by aromatase. Approximately 7% of testosterone is reduced to dihydrotesterone, the more potent testosterone, by 5 alpha-reductase.

9. **A** True

   B False

   C False

   D True

   E True

   The human chorionic gonadotropin (β-hCG) is a glycoprotein composed of 237 amino acids, and it has a molecular mass of 25.7 kDa. The β-hCG promotes the maintenance of the corpus luteum during the beginning of pregnancy. This allows the corpus luteum to secrete the hormone progesterone, thereby making the endometrium lining conducive to pregnancy. The β-hCG is produced by certain gestational trophoblastic tumours.

10. A True

    B True

    C False

    D True

    E False

Hypogonadotrophic hypogonadism is a cause of secondary amenorrhoea. The dysfunction is at the level of the pituitary and hypothalamus and is associated with low follicle-stimulating hormone, luteinising hormone and oestradiol. It can be as a result of stress, exercise, diet or rarely Sheehan's syndrome (pituitary necrosis).

11. A True

    B False

    C False

    D True

    E True

Antidepressants increase prolactin release by inhibiting hypothalamic dopamine secretion, actions which are mediated by the U-receptors. Hyperprolactinaemia has also been noted in patients abusing cocaine. Danazol has an inhibitory effect on LH and FSH. Methyldopa acts through suppression of GnRH related release of FSH and LH.

Chapter 11

Infertility – initial diagnosis

Questions: MCQs

Answer each stem 'True' or 'False'.

1. **Assessment of women presenting with hirsutism:**
    - A Measurement of total testosterone levels represents total androgen load
    - B Free testosterone measurements are more sensitive
    - C There is no need to measure sex hormone binding globulin
    - D There are no clear advantages of measuring levels of serum androstenedione and dehydroepiandrosterone sulfate
    - E Measurement of complete lipid profile

2. **Diagnosis of polycystic ovary syndrome can be made by the following criteria:**
    - A Presence of facial hirsutism
    - B Ultrasound scan showing 8 or more follicles measuring 2–9 mm in diameter
    - C Ovarian volume > 15 mL
    - D Raised free testosterone levels
    - E 17 hydroxyprogesterone levels > 10 ng/mL

3. **With regards to treatment of hirsutism:**
    - A Topical 13.9% eflornithine can be applied on all areas of undesirable hirsutism on a long-term basis
    - B All preparations of combined oral contraceptives can be used for the long term treatment of hirsutism
    - C Third generation pills are superior to combined pills containing desogestrel
    - D Treatment with spironlactone in combination with cyproterone acetate for > 12 months is better than the oral contraceptive alone
    - E Patients being treated with flutamide is very effective long treatment of hirsutism

4. **With regards to unexplained infertility:**
    - A Clomiphene citrate improves pregnancy rates
    - B Intrauterine insemination is an effective treatment of infertility
    - C In vitro fertilisation should be considered for a 35-year-old woman with a history of infertility of 12 months
    - D Intracytoplasmic insemination gives better results than standard in vitro fertilisation in women with unexplained infertility
    - E Ovarian drilling followed by clomiphene citrate stimulation improves pregnancy rates in women with unexplained infertility

5. **With regards to intrauterine pathologies and subfertility:**
   A Intrauterine polypi reduce implantation rates
   B Removal of sub-mucus fibroids improves pregnancy rates
   C Intrauterine synechiae interferes with endometrial growth during ovarian stimulation
   D Hysteroscopic resection of uterine septum should be carried out before assisted conception treatment
   E Hysteroscopic-directed occlusion of the fallopian tubes improves IVF rates in UI

6. **In relation to fallopian tube pathologies and subfertility following are correct:**
   A Women with distal tubal hydrosalpinx should be offered tubal surgery as 40% women will conceive naturally
   B The presence of hydrosalpinx reduces the IVF pregnancy rates
   C Women with tubal disease respond sub optimally to ovarian stimulation
   D Hydrosalpinx should be removed laparoscopically prior to IVF treatment
   E Laparoscopic removal of fallopian tube can decrease ovarian reserve

7. **In the management of ovarian pathologies and assisted conception treatment the following are correct:**
   A In women with polycystic ovaries (PCO), treatment with metformin is as effective as clomiphene citrate
   B In women with PCO, laparoscopic ovarian drilling should always be considered before ovulation induction with clomiphene
   C About 50% of women with stage 2 endometriosis conceive following laparoscopic ablation treatment within 6 months
   D Laparoscopic excision of ovarian endometrioma reduces ovarian reserve
   E IVF pregnancy rates in women with ovarian endometrioma of < 3 cm are similar whether treated or untreated

8. **With regards to ovarian reserve and IVF treatment the following are correct:**
   A Clomiphene citrate challenge test is a good way of assessing ovarian reserve
   B Antimüllerian hormone (AMH) levels assessment is a good predictor of ovarian hyperstimulation
   C Ultrasound assessment of antral follicle count is of value in assessing ovarian reserve
   D AMH levels vary in each cycle
   E Women with a very low AMH level should not be offered assisted conception treatment

9. **Recognised factors for developing ovarian hyperstimulation are:**
   A Women above 40 years
   B Smoking
   C Polycystic ovarian syndrome
   D Using β-hCG for luteal support
   E Obesity

10. Ultrasound diagnosis of a benign ovarian cyst should have following features:

 A Haemorrhagic appearance with peripheral vascularity

 B Papillary structures

 C Very strong blood flow

 D Smooth multilocular with a largest diameter < 100 mm

 E Presence of solid components with the largest component is < 7 mm

Questions: SBAs

11. A 35-year-old woman with known endometriosis has been using progesterone therapy to control her symptoms. Her symptoms have worsened but she is keen to avoid surgery. She is planning to start a monthly gonadotropin-releasing hormone (GnRH) analogue for a course of 6 months. This is her first course of treatment.

    What prescription or investigation should occur alongside this?

    A   Add-back hormone replacement therapy
    B   DEXA scan to assess bone density
    C   Levonorgestrel intrauterine system
    D   No HRT is required
    E   A transvaginal ultrasound scan

12. A 32-year-old woman with known endometriosis has a symptomatic 6 cm endometrioma diagnosed on transvaginal ultrasound scan. Her CA-125 is 157 kU/L. A subsequent MRI scan shows no suspicious features. She has one child and is uncertain about whether her family is complete.

    What is the most appropriate management of her endometrioma?

    A   Drainage of endometrioma and ablation with diathermy
    B   Drainage of endometrioma and vaporisation with CO_2 laser
    C   GnRH analogue with add-back hormone replacement therapy
    D   Ovarian cystectomy
    E   Salpingo-oophorectomy

13. A 45-year-old woman with known endometriosis has a symptomatic 6 cm endometrioma diagnosed on transvaginal ultrasound scan Her CA-125 is 157 kU/L. A subsequent MRI scan shows no suspicious features. She has one child and is certain that her family is complete.

    What is the most appropriate management of her endometrioma?

    A   Drainage of endometrioma and ablation with diathermy
    B   Drainage of endometrioma and vaporisation with CO_2 laser
    C   GnRH analogue with add-back hormone replacement therapy
    D   Ovarian cystectomy
    E   Salpingo-oophorectomy

14. A 40-year-old patient with known endometriosis has dysmenorrhoea, pelvic pain, dyspareunia and menorrhagia. Oral hormonal therapy and the levonorgestrel intrauterine system have been ineffective. She achieved partial symptom relief with GnRH analogues as she became amenorrhoeic. An MRI scan shows a 4 cm endometrioma in the left ovary, a normal right ovary, evidence of thickening of the left uterosacral ligament and diffuse fibroid change within the myometrium (antero-posterior diameter is 10 cm). She is fed up with her symptoms and her family is complete. She comes to you for advice.

What is the most appropriate management to offer her?

A   Bilateral salpingo-oophorectomy
B   Drainage of endometrioma and ablation with diathermy
C   GnRH analogue with add-back hormone replacement therapy
D   Total laparoscopic hysterectomy
E   Total laparoscopic hysterectomy and bilateral salpingo-oophorectomy

15. A 25-year-old patient presents with dysmenorrhoea, pelvic pain and infertility. Her symptoms are gradually worsening and are interfering with her work as a primary school teacher. She is otherwise well, has never been pregnant and has a regular menstrual cycle. She is married and has been trying to conceive for 6 months. Her husband's semen analysis is normal. A clinical examination and transvaginal ultrasound are unremarkable.

What is the most appropriate management?

A   Conservative management
B   Diagnostic laparoscopy only to establish the diagnosis
C   Diagnostic laparoscopy with diathermy or excision of any endometriosis found
D   Laparoscopic ovarian drilling
E   Start GnRH analogues with add-back for 12 months and then start trying for a family

Answers: MCQs

1. A False

    B True

    C False

    E False

    E False

    Measurement of free circulating testosterone is more sensitive than the measurement of total testosterone for the diagnosis of hyperandrogenic disorders. The diagnostic value of total testosterone levels may be enhanced by the concomitant measurement of sex hormone binding globulin. Measurements of androstenedione and dehydroepiandrosterone sulfate concentrations (adrenocortical steroids) may increase the number of subjects identified as hyperandrogenic by 10%.

    A complete evaluation of cardiovascular risk factors such as lipid profile, glucose tolerance and insulin resistance should be restricted to women with obesity, abdominal adiposity and other cardiovascular risk factors.

2. A False

    B False

    C False

    D True

    E False

    An increasing number of women are being diagnosed with polycystic ovary syndrome (PCOS) at ultrasound scanning based on elevated testosterone levels and/ or anovulation, despite not having other hallmarks of PCOS such as hirsutism.

    Ultrasound scan diagnosis is based upon following criteria: presence of either 12 or more follicles measuring 2–9 mm in diameter and/or increased ovarian volume (> 10 mL). It is important to rule out non-classic congenital adrenal hyperplasia by estimation of 17 hydroxyprogesterone.

    Escobar-Morreale HF, Carmina E, Dewailly D, et al. Epidemiology, diagnosis and management of hirsutism: a consensus statement by the Androgen Excess and Polycystic Ovary Syndrome Society. Hum Reprod Update 2012; 18:146–170.

3. A False

    B False

    C False

    D True

    E False

Topical eflornithine is only licensed for facial hirsutism and has not been licensed for the treatment of unwanted terminal hair in areas other than the face. Estrogens in the combined oral contraceptive (COC) pill suppress androgen synthesis and increase levels of sex hormone binding globulin, thereby suppressing levels of free testosterone. Low-dose COC pills, with a progesterone content of either desogestrel, gestodene, cyproterone acetate or drospirenone (spironolactone derivative), are favoured, as these drugs provide normalisation of testosterone levels.

More side effects are reported in third generation COC preparations than second generation preparations. Treatment with spironolactone in combination with cyproterone, finasteride or pills containing cyproterone acetate had better effects than COC pills alone. Flutamide is an antiandrogen and is associated with an increased risk of hepatic toxicity, thus requiring frequent assessment of liver function tests. Patients should also use a reliable form of contraception.

4. A False

    B False

    C False

    D False

    E False

Clomiphene citrate is an antioestrogen and the data from a 2012 randomised trial has not confirmed its superiority in enhancing pregnancy rates in women with unexplained infertility, nor by unstimulated intrauterine insemination, when compared with expectant management. Intracytoplasmic insemination is of proven value for women with male factor infertility. Ovarian drilling is a treatment of choice for women with polycystic ovaries.

5. A True

    B False

    C True

    D False

    E False

A randomised trial has shown has removal of multiple uterine polypi improved pregnancy rates when compared with the control group. A Cochrane review did not report any improvement in pregnancy rates in in vitro fertilisation (IVF) cycles following the treatment of sub mucus fibroids. Presence of intrauterine synechiae per see effects capacity of the uterine cavity and should be treated before considering assisted infertility treatment. Removal of a uterine septum hysteroscopically is not a requirement prior to attempting IVF treatment. Tubal blockage or removal of a fallopian tube should be considered in the presence of hydrosalpinx.

6. A False

    B True

    C False

    D True

    E False

    It has been reported that the fluid within a hydrosalpinx contains substances which are toxic to the embryo, and decrease implantation and pregnancy rates. Therefore, the removal of a diseased fallopian tube improves pregnancy rates. Conservative tubal surgery, on the other hand, increases the risk of an ectopic pregnancy. Salpingectomy does not compromise ovarian reserve. Women with tubal disease respond to ovarian stimulation in same way as those with UI.

7. A False

    B False

    C False

    D True

    E True

    Pregnancy rates following clomiphene treatment in women with PCOS are significantly higher than in women treated with metformin, therefore clomiphene remains the treatment of choice. Ovarian drilling is considered for women who are clomiphene resistant. Laparoscopic surgical excision of stage 1–2 endometriosis is associated with an increased pregnancy rates at 36 weeks, but this association is not seen with laparoscopic ablation. Laparoscopic excision of ovarian endometrioma reduces ovarian reserve. A recent meta-analysis has reported that IVF clinical pregnancy rates per cycle for treated and non-treated small endometrioma groups were comparable.

8. A False

    B True

    C True

    D False

    E False

    The use of clomiphene treatment to assess ovarian reserve is not reliable. Ultrasound assessment of antral follicle count, blood flow and ovarian volume should instead be used to assess ovarian reserve. Antimüllerian hormone (AMH) and antral follicle count are reliable predictors of ovarian response to ovarian hyperstimulation. AMH levels do not fluctuate during menstrual cycles. Women with low AMH can be managed by special stimulation regimens during IVF treatment and pregnancies have been reported.

9. A False

   B False

   C True

   D False

   E False

Risk factors for the development of ovarian hyperstimulation are: young age, low body weight, PCOS, higher doses of exogenous gonadotrophin used, large number of follicles, rapidly rising oestradiol levels and β-hCG trigger for ovulation.

10. A True

    B False

    C False

    D True

    E True

The International Ovarian Tumour Analysis (IOTA) group has standardised the descriptive terms used in ultrasound scanning of adnexal lesions:

- Benign masses are: unilocular cysts, presence of solid components where the largest component is <7 mm, presence of acoustic shadowing, smooth multilocular tumours with a largest diameter <100 mm and no blood flow
- Malignant masses are: irregular solid tumour, ascites, at least 4 papillary structures, irregular multilocular solid tumour with largest diameter >100 mm and very strong blood flow

Answers: SBAs

11. A Add-back hormone replacement therapy

It is generally recommended to prescribe hormonal add-back therapy to coincide with the start of GnRH agonist therapy, to prevent bone loss and hypoestrogenic symptoms during treatment. Add-back estrogen therapy is not known to reduce the effect of treatment on pain relief.

12. D Ovarian cystectomy

In a woman with endometrioma, cystectomy (not drainage and coagulation) is indicated because it reduces endometriosis-associated pain.

13. E Salpingo-oophorectomy

Although European Society of Human Reproduction and Embryology guidelines suggest ovarian cystectomy, it would be more sensible to consider an oophorectomy due to her small risk of malignancy. The size of the endometrioma may leave very little functional tissue behind and her family is complete. Oophorectomy is the safer option in this situation.

14. E Total laparoscopic hysterectomy and bilateral salpingo-oophorectomy

In a woman who has completed her family and failed to respond to conservative treatments, hysterectomy with removal of ovaries and all visible endometriotic lesions should be considered. Hysterectomy will not necessarily cure symptoms or disease.

15. C Diagnostic laparoscopy with diathermy or excision of any endometriosis found

In women with AFS/ASRM stage I/II endometriosis, operative laparoscopy (to excise or ablate endometriosis lesion) with adhesiolysis rather than diagnostic laparoscopy is recommended because operative laparoscopy is associated with an increased pregnancy rate.

Chapter 12

Endometriosis

Questions: MCQs

Answer each stem 'True' or 'False'.

1. **Regarding endometriosis presentation:**
   A The prevalence of endometriosis in the general population is 2–10%
   B The prevalence of endometriosis in infertile women is 70% 50%
   C The overall diagnostic delay in the UK is 4 years 8YB
   D Dysmenorrhea is the chief complaint in 90% of patients with endometriosis
   E Pain is referred to legs and back in adolescents with endometriosis in 31% of cases

2. **When compared with controls, women with endometriosis have odds ratios [OR (95% CI)] for the following symptoms:**
   A Abdominopelvic pain 5.2 (4.7–5.7)
   B Dysmenorrhea 8.1 (7.2–9.3)
   C Heavy menstrual bleeding 1.8 (1.2–2.5)
   D Infertility 8.2 (6.9–9.9)
   E Dyspareunia/postcoital bleeding 6.8 (5.7–8.2)

3. **When diagnosing endometriosis:**
   A Transvaginal ultrasound is more useful than MRI for the diagnosis of rectovaginal disease
   B Ground glass echogenicity, one to four compartments and no papillary structures with detectable blood flow are the characteristic features of an endometrioma on trans-vaginal scan
   C A diagnostic laparoscopy is the gold standard for diagnosis
   D It is essential to obtain histological confirmation of the disease
   E A raised CA-125 is diagnostic of endometriosis

4. **Regarding the surgical management of endometriosis:**
   A Endometriosis seen at diagnostic laparoscopy should not be treated until a trial of medical therapy has been completed
   B Clinicians should only consider excision of peritoneal disease to reduce pain symptoms
   C When managing endometriomas surgically they should always be drained & coagulated and medical treatment started to reduce endometriosis symptoms
   D Only peritoneal disease should be treated surgically. Deep infiltrating endometriosis is best treated with medical therapy such as GnRH analogues

E Patients with suspected or diagnosed deep endometriosis should be referred to a centre of expertise that offers all available treatments in a multidisciplinary context

5. **Regarding perioperative medical therapy for endometriosis:**

A All patients should receive hormonal therapy preoperatively as this improves the outcome of surgery with respect to pain

B All patients should receive hormonal therapy postoperatively as this improves the outcome of surgery with respect to pain

C All patients who have had an ovarian cystectomy for an ovarian endometrioma and are not immediately seeking conception should be offered hormonal contraceptives

D Postoperative use of a levonorgestrel-releasing intrauterine system or a combined hormonal contraceptive for at least 18–24 months helps prevent secondary endometriosis associated dysmenorrhoea

E Surgical management of endometriosis should always be followed by at least 3 months of medical therapy

Questions: EMQs

Questions 6 – 10

Options for Questions 6 – 10:

A   Combined oral contraceptive pill
B   Bilateral salpingo-oophorectomy
C   Diagnostic laparoscopy
D   GnRH analogue
E   GnRH analogue + add-back hormone
   replacement therapy
F   Hysterectomy
G   Hysterectomy and bilateral salpingo-
   oophorectomy
H   Levonorgestrel intrauterine system
   (insert or replace)

I   None of the above
J   Pain team referral
K   Pelvic MRI
L   Pelvic ultrasound scan
M   Progesterone-only pill/depot medroxy
   progesterone acetate
N   Referral to another specialty
O   Tricycling combined oral
   contraceptive pill

For each clinical scenario described below, choose the next most appropriate
intervention from the list of options above. Each option may be used once, more than
once or not at all.

6. A 25-year-old patient with a body mass index of 26 is referred by her general
practitioner with a 3-year history of dysmenorrhoea, non-menstrual pelvic pain
and dyspareunia. She has been tri-cycling her COCP, which she is reliant upon
for contraception, for 9 months. Despite this she reports that her symptoms are
worsening. She has no significant past medical or surgical history and her clinical
examination is unremarkable other than bilateral adnexal tenderness.

7. A 30-year-old patient with known endometriosis comes to clinic for review. She is
using a levonorgestrel intrauterine system for both endometriosis management
and contraception. It was inserted 4 years ago. She has on-going problems with
non-menstrual pelvic pain associated with abdominal bloating. This tends to be
associated with bouts of constipation. She reports no loss of blood or mucus from
her back passage.

8. A 45-year-old woman with known endometriosis has been managing her disease
with a GnRH analogue and tibolone. She is para 2 and her husband has had a
vasectomy. Her symptoms are well controlled but she is fed up with monthly
injections and requests a hysterectomy.

9. A 22-year-old woman presents with symptoms suggestive of endometriosis.
She uses inhalers for asthma and has no surgical history. She has just started a
relationship and is currently using condoms for contraception. At her diagnostic
laparoscopy mild endometriosis was noted in the left ovarian fossa and over the
right side of the uterovesical fold. This was treated with diathermy.

10. A 28-year-old woman had endometriosis confirmed at diagnostic laparoscopy
2 years ago. She had diathermy treatment and changed from the COCP to POP.

Her symptoms were well controlled for about a year but over the last 6 months have worsened considerably. She has pain most days and has had to take a week off work with her period for the last 2 months. She is fed up with her symptoms as they are interfering with her life. She has no immediate plans for a family at this time.

Questions 11 – 14

Options for question 11 – 14:

A Combined oral contraceptive pill
B Bilateral salpingo-oophorectomy
C Diagnostic laparoscopy
D GnRH analogue
E GnRH analogue + add-back hormone
    replacement therapy
F Hysterectomy
G Hysterectomy and bilateral salpingo-
    oophorectomy
H Levonorgestrel intrauterine system
    (insert or replace)

I Pain team referral
J Pelvic CT/MRI
K Pelvic ultrasound scan
L Progesterone-only pill/depot medroxy
    progesterone acetate
M Referral to another specialty
N Tricycling combined oral
    contraceptive pill
O None of the above

For each clinical scenario described below, choose the single most appropriate next step in managing the patient's disease from the list of options above. Each option may be used once, more than once or not at all.

11. A 32-year-old woman with known endometriosis undergoes laparoscopy to assess her disease because she is struggling with significant pelvic pain and dyspareunia despite GnRH analogues and add-back HRT. At surgery a nodule is palpable in the posterior fornix and the pouch of Douglas is seen to be partially obliterated with significant disease over both uterosacral ligaments.

12. A 43-year-old woman with known endometriosis underwent a repeat laparoscopy to re-evaluate her disease. She uses a levonorgestrel intrauterine system for contraception and has been experiencing pelvic pain, dyspareunia, dyschezia and cyclical rectal bleeding. At laparoscopy a large nodule of deep infiltrating endometriosis is seen overlying the rectum and appears to be tethered to the underlying muscularis.

13. A 25-year-old woman with a BMI of 26 is referred by her general practitioner with a 3-year history of dysmenorrhoea, non-menstrual pelvic pain and dyspareunia. She has been tri-cycling her COCP, which she is reliant upon for contraception, for 9 months. Despite this she reports her symptoms are worsening. She has no significant past medical or surgical history. Clinical examination reveals a left adnexal swelling that is tender and some induration of the left uterosacral ligament.

14. A 25-year-old woman is managing her endometriosis with the progesterone only pill. She is amenorrhoeic and is much happier with her symptoms but still has flares of pelvic pain. There does not seem to be a particular pattern nor are there triggers. She cannot tolerate non-steroidal anti-inflammatory drugs and finds codeine causes constipation.

Answers: MCQs

1. A True

   B False

   C False

   D False

   E True

   The prevalence of endometriosis in infertile women is 50%. The overall diagnostic delay varies between countries; in the UK it is 8 years. 62% of women complained of dysmenorrhoea in a Brazilian study.

2. A True

   B True

   C False

   D True

   E True

   The odds ratio for heavy menstrual bleeding is 4.0 (3.5–4.5).

3. A False

   B True

   C True

   D False

   E False

   It is a good practice point to obtain histological confirmation of disease but it is not essential for diagnosis. CA-125 is often elevated in endometriosis but this has no diagnostic value. MRI is the modality of choice for investigating rectovaginal disease but a transvaginal scan is appropriate for other pelvic endometriosis and endometriomas.

4. A False

   B False

   C False

   D False

   E True

   When endometriosis is diagnosed at laparoscopy, surgical management is recommended to reduce the associated pain. Ablation and excision of peritoneal endometriosis to reduce endometriosis-associated pain may be considered.

When performing surgery in women with ovarian endometrioma, only cystectomy should be performed, as it reduces pain. Drainage and coagulation maybe considered when the endometrioma is very large or risk of oophorectomy is high, however this may reduce ovarian reserve.

Surgical removal of deep endometrioma may be considered as it reduces endometriosis-associated pain.

5. A **False**

    B **False**

    C **True**

    D **True**

    E **False**

Preoperative hormonal treatment should not be prescribed to improve the outcome of surgery for pain in women with endometriosis. Adjunctive hormonal treatment is also ineffective in reducing endometriosis-associated pain after surgery. After a cystectomy for ovarian endometrioma in women not immediately seeking conception, hormonal contraceptives are recommended for the secondary prevention of endometrioma.

For the postoperative secondary prevention of endometriosis-associated dysmenorrhea in women who have been operated on for endometriosis, a levonorgestrel-releasing intrauterine system or a combined hormonal contraceptive for at least 18–24 months is advised. This approach is not advised for non-menstrual pelvic pain or dyspareunia, however.

In patients where fertility is concerned, there is no evidence to support postoperative medical therapy, therefore these patients should be advised to conceive as soon as they feel ready.

Answers: EMQs

6. C Diagnostic laparoscopy

This patient has a 3-year history and has tried first line medical therapy for 9 months without relief of her symptoms. The next step is to establish a diagnosis with a diagnostic laparoscopy.

7. N Referral to another specialty

A history of pain, bloating and constipation are suggestive of irritable bowel syndrome and referral to gastroenterology would be reasonable. Her levonorgestrel releasing intrauterine system will need changing in 1 year but will provide contraception cover for a further year.

8. B Bilateral salpingo-oophorectomy

Definitive surgical management for this patient would be a bilateral salpingo-oophorectomy. There is no indication to do a hysterectomy, which carries extra risks.

9. M Progesterone-only pill/depot medroxy progesterone acetate

The disease is mild and has been heat treated. It would be reasonable to suggest on-going medical therapy and her current method of contraception is less reliable than the progesterone-only pill or depot medroxy progesterone acetate. It is important to consider this patient's contraceptive needs as well as the diagnosis or endometriosis.

10. E GnRH analogue + add-back hormone replacement therapy

It would be reasonable to pursue more aggressive medical therapy to control her symptoms. This should be used with add-back therapy to minimise side effects.

11. K Pelvic ultrasound scan

This patient is likely to have deep infiltrating disease that will require surgical excision. To plan this and to evaluate the rectovaginal septum an MRI is required.

12. N Tricycling combined oral contraceptive pill

In this situation it would be sensible to refer this patient to a colorectal surgeon or to a specialist centre for a possible rectal shave or disc resection.

13. L Progesterone-only pill/depot medroxy progesterone acetate

The patient has a 3-year history and has tried first line medical therapy for 9 months without relief of her symptoms. The next step is to establish a diagnosis but imaging to assess her left adnexa is the next step to allow surgical planning – possible ovarian cystectomy.

14. J Pelvic CT/MRI

The hormonal therapy is probably appropriate but the patient is struggling with her analgesia. A referral to the pain team would be helpful.

07760707908

Chapter 13

Preventative gynaecology

Questions: MCQs

Answer each stem 'True' or 'False'.

1. **Regarding vulvodynia:**
   A Vulvodynia has been described as a neuropathic pain disorder
   B It is more common among white American women than Hispanic
   C Most women with vulvodynia complain of a burning pain at physical examination of the vagina
   D Women should be screened for candidiasis
   E Topical application of Lidocaine gel is more effective palliative measure as compared with topical nitro-glycerine gel for coital activity

2. **Regarding pruritus vulvae:**
   A The sensations are transmitted by B fibres to the spinothalamic tract via the dorsal horn of the spinal cord
   B Pruritus is exacerbated by hot ambient conditions
   C Cytokines are involved in atopic vulvitis
   D Serotonins mediated mechanism is involved in herpes simplex
   E Histamine released by mast cells is involved in polycythaemia vera

3. **Regarding lichen sclerosus:**
   A It is an auto immune disorder with malignant potential
   B It affects women of all age groups
   C Thyroid disease is more frequent in patients with LS than the control
   D The lesions are well-delimited red erosive located on the inner side of labia minora
   E Histological diagnosis should always be made before starting any treatment

4. **The following conditions should be suspected in patients with persistent pruritus vulvae despite treatment with ultra-potent steroids:**
   A Vulvodynia
   B Squamous cell carcinoma
   C Contact dermatitis
   D Acanthotic areas
   E Well-differentiated vulval intraepithelial neoplasia

5. In differential diagnosis of vulval lesions:

    A   Chronic erosions are seen in vulval intraepithelial neoplasia
    B   Red Patches are seen in squamous cell carcinoma
    C   White patches are seen in lichen sclerosus
    D   Hypertrophic patches are seen in Zoon's vulvitis
    E   Vulvovaginal-gingival syndrome is seen in lichen planus

6. Regarding lichen planus:

    A   Women usually presents with dyspareunia
    B   Lichen planus may be asymptomatic
    C   Red erosive lesions are usually located on the vestibule
    D   Erosive lichen planus may present with frontal scarring alopecia
    E   Malignant transformation to squamous cell carcinoma is likely

Answers: MCQs

1. A True

    B False

    C True

    D True

    E True

    Vulvodynia is a complex disorder of multiple aetiologies but the most compelling origin is a neuropathic disorder. It is more common in Hispanic women than in white Americans or Africans. Most women with vulvodynia complain of provoked or unprovoked pain with a physical contact to the vaginal canal (examination, attempted intercourse and even insertion of a tampon). The pain can be constant or intermittent.

    A detailed history should be taken to rule out a sexually-transmitted disease and any suggestion of chemical contact dermatitis. One study has reported a high incidence on *Candida* infection in this group of women. Topical application of lidocaine around the vaginal orifice on a long-term basis facilitates intercourse in up to 50% women. Nitroglycerine gel is another option but its side effects limit its use.

2. A False

    B True

    C True

    D False

    E False

    The sensations are transmitted by C fibres, not by B fibres. Scratch sensation is an innate deep reflex. Pruritus is exacerbated by skin inflammation, dry or hot ambient conditions, skin vasodilatation, and psychological stressors. Histamine is released by mast cells in allergic dermatitis. Cytokines and immune-mediated pro-inflammatory agents are involved in atopic vulvitis; nerve paraesthesia in herpes simplex and serotonin-mediated pruritus occurs in polycythaemia vera, uraemia, cholestasis and lymphoma.

3. A False

    B True

    C True

    D False

    E False

    Lichen sclerosus (LS) is a chronic non-neoplastic, non-infectious, inflammatory skin disorder affecting the genital area. It is considered an auto-immune disorder, occurring in genetically predisposed individuals. In one study, thyroid disease was more frequent in women with LS than other conditions such as alopecia areata, morphea and pernicious anaemia. LS lesions are pallor and it may be widespread and scarring resulting from adhesions from synechiae between two contiguous surfaces involved by LS. Histological diagnosis is not required before staring treatment with strong steroids locally.

4. A True

    B True

    C True

    D True

    E True

All these causes are correct. Resistance to steroids is another unusual cause.

5. A False

    B False

    C True

    D False

    E True

Chronic erosions are seen with Paget's disease, squamous cell carcinoma (SCC) and mucus membrane pemphigoid. Red patches are seen with Zoon's vulvitis, vulval intraepithelial neoplasia (VIN) and Paget's disease. White patches are seen with lichen sclerosus, and hypertrophic patches are in VIN and SCC.

6. A True

    B True

    C True

    D True

    E False

Lichen planus may be asymptomatic or responsible for soreness, burning, pruritus or dyspareunia. The morphological features can be divided into three categories: erosive, atrophic or hypertrophic. Erosive lichen planus is a multicentric condition which may have serious consequences for quality of life. The lesions consist of well-delimited red erosive or atrophic areas mainly located on the vestibule, the inner side of labia minora and the clitoris. Erosive lichen planus may present with frontal alopecia in 50% cases. Malignant transformation has been reported but it is rare.

Chapter 14

Adolescent gynaecology

Questions: MCQs

Answer each stem 'True' or 'False'.

1. **Primary amenorrhoea**

   An 18-year-old girl has presented with total absence of periods. This is caused by:

   ×A   Mosaic Turner's syndrome
   ✓B   Pure gonadal dysgenesis
   ✓C   Empty sella turcica syndrome
   ✓D   Methyldopa
   ✓E   Cranial irradiation

2. **Assessment of women with primary amenorrhoea should include:**

   ✓A   Estimation of follicle-stimulation hormone (FSH) levels
   ✓B   Estimation of serum levels of testosterone
   ✓C   Chromosomal analysis
   ✓D   Assessment of body mass index
   ✓E   Estimation of thyroid function test

3. **Regarding Turner syndrome:**

   ×A   It is associated with 45 XO/XX
   ×B   The incidence is 1:1500
   ✓C   The missing gene on the X-chromosome is the short-stature homeobox gene
   ×D   Women have normal height for their age
   ✓E   Gonadotrophin levels are lower than normal

4. **Regarding pure gonadal dysgenesis:**

   ×A   Their chromosomal pattern is 46 XY
   +B   Ovaries have reduced ovarian follicles numbers
   ×C   Follicle-stimulating hormone levels are elevated
   +D   Combined hormone replacement therapy treatment can successfully induce ovulation
   ✓E   Up to 10% women conceive spontaneously

5. **Regarding Mayer–Rokitansky–Küster–Hauser syndrome:**

   ×A   Its incidence is 1 in 20,000   1:5000
   ✓B   It is caused by an inherited gene defect
   ×C   Patient has a normal vagina

+D   Uterus is of normal shape and fully developed

E   The ovarian development may be normal

6.   **Regarding primary amenorrhea and androgen insensitivity syndrome:**

A   Its incidence is 1 in 20,000

B   It is caused by a mutation in the androgen receptor gene

C   The affected individuals have 46 XY chromosomes

D   Secondary sexual characteristics are poorly developed

E   They may require genital reconstructive surgery

7.   **Primary amenorrhea is caused by the following:**

A   Excessive exercise

B   Severe stress

C   Craniopharyngioma

D   Wegner's granulomatosis

E   Kallmann's syndrome

Questions: SBAs

For each question, select the single best answer from the five options listed.

8. An 18-year-old girl has presented with abnormal vaginal discharge. Cultures of the purulent discharge confirm *Neisseria gonorrhoea* and *Chlamydia trachomatis* co-infection.

    What is the most cost-effective treatment?

    A   Azithromycin 1 g per os one dose
    B   Ceftriaxone 500 mg intramuscular + azithromycin 1 g per os one dose
    C   Ceftriaxone 500 mg intramuscular + doxycycline 100 mg twice daily for 7 days
    D   Doxycycline 100 mg twice daily for 7 days
    E   Ofloxacin 200 mg twice daily or 400 mg once daily for 7 days

9. A 16-year-old girl presents to the gynaecology outpatient clinic with primary amenorrhoea. Her breast development is Tanner stage IV. She has a blind vaginal pouch and no cervix.

    Which of the following describes the most likely diagnosis?

    A   Gonadal dysgenesis
    B   Kallman's syndrome
    C   Late onset congenital adrenal hyperplasia
    D   Mayer–Rokitansky–Küster–Hauser syndrome
    E   Polycystic ovarian syndrome

Answers: MCQs

1. A False

    B True

    C True

    D True

    E True

    Turner syndrome is diagnosed by a karyotype of 45 XO whereas in mosaicism, the X-chromosome is missing in some cells. Some women with this condition will reach puberty and menstruate but suffer from early secondary amenorrhea. Gonadal dysgenesis is associated with accelerated loss of germ cells in utero and hence hormonal failure. Such women present with sexual infantilism and infertility. Empty Sella syndrome sometime causes hyperprolactinaemia. This condition may be primary or secondary to injury or radiation. Methyldopa also causes hyperprolactinaemia, hence amenorrhoea.

2. A True

    B True

    C True

    D True

    E True

    Follicle-stimulation hormone levels will be elevated in women with primary ovarian failure and pure gonadal dysgenesis. Lower levels will be seen in patients with pan hypopituitarism.

    An elevated level of testosterone is associated with polycystic syndrome.

    Chromosomal analysis is required to rule out androgen insensitivity syndrome and Turner's syndrome.

    A very low body mass index is associated with anorexia nervosa and absence of menstruation. Abnormal thyroid function test helps to diagnose thyroid disease and even direct towards a possible hyperprolactinaemia.

3. A False

    B False

    C True

    D False

    E True

    These women have normal 46 XX chromosomes. More than 60% women have undetectable ovaries with no follicular growth, thus leading to high levels of follicle-stimulating hormone. The estrogen component of hormone replacement therapy helps to develop secondary sexual characteristics, followed by initiation of menstruation. Progesterone protects against endometrial hyperplasia. Majority of these women will require oocyte-donated in vitro fertilisation treatment for their infertility, but 5–10% women have sporadic ovulation and can conceive naturally.

4. A False

B False

C False

D False

E True

This occurs in about 1 in 5000 cases. It is caused by sporadic genetic mutations affecting Müllerian differentiation during intrauterine development. These women have an absent upper one-third of vagina and a hypoplastic uterus. The first line of treatment is to advice on measures for progressive vaginal dilatation. The ovarian development is unaffected as it develops from mesoderm.

5. A False

B True

C False

D False

E True

Population-based studies estimate a prevalence about 1 in 5000 live female births. Atypical cases of Mayer–Rokitansky–Küster–Hauser (MRKH) syndrome can be associated with genetic mutation. A genetic mutation causes a leucine-to-proline residue substitution at amino acid position 12. It is also reported that this is associated with a deletion mutation in chromosome 17.

MRKH syndrome is also typically associated with complete or partial absence of uterus and cervix. The vagina is very shortened or absent. Intercourse may be very painful or impossible. The diagnosis is made at puberty when the patient presents with primary amenorrhoea with normal secondary sexual characteristics. The patient's chromosome constellation will be 46 XX.

6. A False

B True

C True

D False

E True

The incidence of androgen-insensitivity syndrome (AIS) is around 1 in 60,000. It is caused by a mutation in the androgen receptor gene which may lead to partial or complete AIS. The affected individuals have 46 XY with a female phenotype. The gonads (testicular tissue) are usually intra-abdominal or in the inguinal region.

Due to partial or total lack of binding with androgen receptors, these individuals may have some or no androgenisation. However, because of peripheral aromatisation of testosterone to estrogens, secondary sexual characteristics are well developed. If these individuals have been brought up as females, then gender assignment surgery is required.

7. A True

    B True

    C True

    D True

    E True

There appears to be a chronic imbalance between caloric intake and consumption among high performance athletes, and it leads to hypothalamic dysfunction. Severe stress leads to raised levels of corticotrophin releasing hormone which inhibits gonadotropin-releasing hormone (GnRH) pulsatility, thus leading to amenorrhea. Space-occupying lesions, like craniopharyngioma and glioma, act by interfering with the normal pulsatility of GnRH (local compression or destructive effect). Wegner's granulomatosis is an infiltrative disorder of hypothalamus. Kallmann's syndrome is characterised by complete or partial absence of smell. There is disrupted migration of GnRH producing nerve cells in the brain.

Answers: SBAs

8. B Ceftriaxone 500 mg IM + azithromycin 1 g PO one dose

The British Association of Sexual Health and HIV (BASHH) recommends treatment for uncomplicated *Neisseria gonorrhoeae* infection with ceftriaxone 500 mg given intramuscularly with 1 g of azithromycin. The azithromycin is given as an adjunct treatment to protect the ceftriaxone in order to delay the development of resistance and not to treat co-existing chlamydia, although it will also do this. It should be noted however, that because *N. gonorrhoeae* exhibits significant tetracycline resistance, doxycycline should not be used in place of azithromycin. Ofloxacin has similar efficacy to doxycycline but carries a risk of *Clostridium difficile* infection and tendon rupture. It is also considerably more expensive than doxycycline.

9. D Mayer–Rokitansky–Küster–Hauser syndrome

Normal breast development with no cervix or uterus and a blind vaginal pouch may be caused by either Müllerian agenesis or androgen insensitivity. Kallmann's syndrome is associated with delayed puberty (Tanner stage I breasts).

Chapter 15

Benign outpatient gynaecology

Questions: SBAs

For each question, select the single best answer from the five options listed.

1. A 48-year-old multiparous woman presents with heavy menstrual bleeding. Her ultrasound scan is normal.

   What should the next step in her management be?

   A Hysteroscopy
   B Hysterectomy
   C Endometrial biopsy
   D Reassure
   E Gonadotropin-releasing hormone analogues

2. Tranexamic acid belongs to one of the following groups:

   A COX inhibitor
   B COX activator
   C Antifibrinolytic
   D Plasminogen activator
   E Menstrual endometrium stabiliser

3. A 31-year-old woman had a large loop excision of the transformation zone (LLETZ) for high grade abnormality of her cervix 3 months ago.

   What is the most appropriate follow up?

   A Colposcopy 6 months following LLETZ
   B Colposcopy and treatment 6 months from LLETZ
   C Human papilloma virus (HPV) blood test at 6 months
   D Smear and HPV testing at a general practice 6-months post LLETZ
   E Smear and HPV testing at a general practice 12 months following LLETZ

4. **A 54-year-old woman presents to the general gynaecology clinic with an incidental finding of a 4 cm simple right ovarian cyst. Her CA-125 is 24 kU/L.**

   What is the best option for her?

   A   Recommend an exploratory laparotomy
   B   Recommend a laparoscopic bilateral salpingo-oophorectomy
   C   Recommend an ovarian cystectomy
   D   Refer to a gynaecological oncologist
   E   Repeat the pelvic ultrasound and CA-125 in 4 months

5. **Which of the following findings on transvaginal scan is a definitive of the diagnosis of missed miscarriage?**

   A   Crown–rump length of 3.4 mm with no fetal heart
   B   Crown–rump length of 6.7 mm with no fetal heart
   C   Crown–rump length of 8.6 mm with no fetal heart
   D   Empty gestational sac with a mean sac diameter of 15 mm
   E   Gestational sac with mean sac diameter of 19 mm, with presence of yolk sac but no fetal pole

6. **Methotrexate can be offered as the first line treatment for ectopic pregnancy in which of the following scenarios?**

   A   Stable patient with β-human chorionic gonadotropin (β-hCG) of 348 IU/L with significant amount of echogenic fluid in the abdomen
   B   Stable patient with β-hCG of 6648 IU/L
   C   Stable patient with a live ectopic pregnancy (fetal heart seen)
   D   Stable patient with β-hCG of 1487 IU/L and minimal free fluid in the pouch of Douglas (POD)
   E   Stable patient with β-hCG of 4487 IU/L and minimal free fluid in the POD

7. **A 32-year-old nulliparous woman presents with heavy menstrual bleeding. Ultrasound scan shows a grade 0 submucosal fibroid of 5 cm. The patient is keen to have children.**

   What management option are you most likely to consider for her?

   A   A levonorgestrel-releasing intrauterine system
   B   Hysteroscopic fibroid resection
   C   Uterine artery embolisation
   D   GnRH analogues
   E   Hysterectomy

8. **A 40-year-old woman presents with cyclical mood swings and abdominal bloating in the premenstrual phase of the menstrual cycle.**

   Which of these these modalities of treatment will you not consider?

   A   GnRH analogues
   B   Contraceptive pill

C Laparoscopic bilateral oophorectomy

D Cyclical progestogens

E Antidepressants

9. A 24-year-old woman is diagnosed with an ectopic pregnancy on ultrasound. Her serum β-hCG level measured on the day was 1100 mIU/mL and she was given 50 mg/m² of methotrexate intramuscularly. Five days later, she complains of increased lower abdominal pain. Her blood pressure is 120/78 mmHg and pulse is 78 beats per minute. Her abdomen shows some tenderness in the left iliac fossa with no guarding or rebound.

Which of the following is the best course of action?

A Laparoscopy +/– salpingectomy

B Laparotomy

C Repeat dose of methotrexate

D Repeat serum β-hCG level

E Repeat ultrasound scan

10. A 37-year-old woman presented with vaginal spotting at 7 weeks' gestation. Transabdominal ultrasound scan suggests a mean sac diameter of 24 mm with no fetal pole seen.

What is the most appropriate course of action?

A Repeat ultrasound scan in 2 weeks

B Transvaginal scan in 2 weeks

C Perform transvaginal scan at same setting

D Measure serum β-hCG

E Offer medical management of miscarriage

11. Which of the following management options for a miscarriage are associated with reduced rate of fever and rigors, and improved patient satisfaction?

A Misoprostol 400 μg oral

B Misoprostol 400 μg rectal

C Misoprostol 400 μg vaginal

D Misoprostol 800 μg oral

E Misoprostol 800 μg vaginal

12. A 65-year-old woman presented with an episode of post-menopausal bleeding lasting one week. An outpatient hysteroscopy finds a 3 cm endometrial polyp.

What would be your next line of management?

A Blind avulsion of the polyp in the outpatient clinic

B Endometrial biopsy

C Hysterectomy

D Hysteroscopic resection of polyp under general anaesthetic

E Repeat outpatient hysteroscopy in 6 months

Questions: EMQs

Questions 13 – 17

Option list for Questions 13 – 17:

A   Adenomyosis
B   Chronic pelvic pain
C   Endometriosis
D   Endosalpingiosis
E   Inflammatory bowel syndrome
F   Hydrosalpinx
G   Leiomyoma
H   Ovarian cyst

I   Pelvic congestion
J   Pelvic inflammatory disease
K   Primary dysmenorrhoea
L   Secondary dysmenorrhoea (70–80%, pre-menstrual ache, spasmodic dysmenorrhoea, decreases as bleeding slows)
M   None of the above

For each of the following cases, select the single most appropriate diagnosis from the list above. Each option may be used once, more than once or not at all.

13. A 18-year-old woman is referred to the hospital with pelvic pain as the general practitioner suspects endometriosis. She started her periods at the age of 12 and they are regular. She has always had some mild dysmenorrhoea but is now getting much more non-menstrual pelvic pain. On questioning she reports deep dyspareunia with her current partner but reports no problems with her previous sexual partners.

14. A 24-year-old patient undergoes a diagnostic laparoscopy for pelvic pain. There are clear nodules noted on the pelvic side wall and these are biopsied. They are reported as originating from the fallopian tube.

15. A 28-year-old patient presents to her general practitioner with primary infertility and intermittent pelvic pain. She has been trying for 2 years but has never conceived. She has no significant past medical history other than being treated for chlamydia 5 years ago. Her partner's semen analysis is normal and her general practitioner arrangs an ultrasound. On ultrasound a large cystic swelling is noted in the left adnexa. The left ovary is seen separate from this and contains a small functional cyst.

16. A 40-year-old patient presents with dysmenorrhoea and menorrhagia. Upon being questioned she reports intermittent dyspareunia that is positional but no real pelvic pain through the rest of her cycle. She is para 2 and has completed her family. On examination the uterus feels diffusely enlarged and is quite tender to palpate.

17. A 22-year-old patient is referred to the general surgeons with suspected appendicitis. She has a 2-month history of right–sided pelvic pain but it has been much worse in the last 48 hours. She is not in a relationship, having split up with her boyfriend 6 months ago. She has mildly raised inflammatory markers. A diagnostic laparoscopy is performed. During the laparoscopy the surgeons ask for a gynaecological opinion, as the abdomen and pelvis appear entirely normal. A specimen of peritoneal fluid is sent for microbiological assessment but no organisms are grown.

Questions 18 – 21

Option list for Questions 18 – 21

A Corpus luteal cyst	H Ovarian torsion
B Endometrioma	I Pelvic inflammatory disease
C Granulosa cell tumour	J Polycystic ovaries
D Haemorrhagic cyst	K Ruptured ovarian cyst
E Mature cystic ovarian teratoma	L Thecoma
F Ovarian epithelial tumour	M Tubo-ovarian abscess
G Ovarian fibroma	

For each of the following cases, select the single most likely diagnosis from the list above. Each option may be used once, more than once or not at all.

18. A 32-year-old woman presents to the rapid access clinic, referred by her general practitioner with pelvic pain and dysmenorrhea. She has had the pain for many years but her general practitioner only recently organised a pelvic scan and blood test. Her CA-125 is 2230 kU/L and the ultrasound scan reveals bilateral enlarged ovaries containing diffuse low level echoes and a single thick septation. There is no colour flow and no free fluid.

19. A 28-year-old woman presents with severe abdominal pain and offensive discharge and pyrexia of 38.3°C. She had a coil put in for contraception 3 months ago. A pelvic ultrasound revealed bilateral thick walled multilocular cystic lesions continuous with the fallopian tube. There is moderate free fluid in the pouch of Douglas.

20. A 36-year-old woman has a pelvic scan as part of her fertility work up. She is asymptomatic. The scan reveals bilateral ovarian complex masses that contain both solid and cystic components. The right ovary contains a cystic mass with a solid, highly echogenic 'dermoid plug'. Her CA-125 is 15 kU/L.

21. A 19-year-old woman presents to emergency department with acute onset severe lower abdominal pain. A pelvic ultrasound reveals a 7 cm ovarian cyst on the left ovary with a thin wall and reticular pattern, there is no internal blood flow. There is a small amount of free fluid in the pouch of Douglas. The emergency department has requested a CA-125 but the result is not back yet.

Questions 22 – 23

Option list for Questions 22 – 23:

A   Myomectomy

B   Hysterectomy

C   GnRH analogues

D   Hysteroscopic resection of submucous fibroid

E   Fibroid embolisation

G   Ulipristal acetate

H   A levonorgestrel-releasing intrauterine system

I   Tranexamic acid

For each case described below, choose the single most likely management option from the above list of options. Each option may be used once, more than once, or not at all.

22. A 43-year-old mother of two is known to have uterine fibroids and menorrhagia for many years. In the past she has responded well to tranexamic acid and a levonorgestrel-releasing intrauterine system, but she has noticed that her bleeding is getting heavier and she feels exhausted. She also complains of feeling bloated, abdominal pain and constipation, as new symptoms. You are seeing her with a scan report that confirms the presence of multiple uterine fibroids with largest one measuring $15 \times 10 \times 18$ cm in the posterior uterine wall.

23. A 48-year-old nulliparous Afro-Caribbean woman is referred by her general practitioner (GP) complaining of heavy menstrual loss for the last 3 months. She is known to have had three small intramural fibroids since she was 27 years of age. Her periods have always been heavy, but for the last 3 months she has been passing clots during the first 3–4 days of her cycle. The GP has requested a pelvic scan for her and there is no significant change in the size of fibroids: the largest still measures 4×5 cm.

Questions 24 – 25

Option list for Questions 24 – 25:

A Mefenamic acid and tranexamic acid   E Endometrial ablation
B A levonorgestrel-releasing intrauterine   F GnRH analogues
   system   G Hysterectomy
C Hysteroscopy   H Uterine artery embolisation
D Endometrial biopsy   I Hysteroscopic fibroid resection

For each case described below, choose the single most likely management option from the above list of options. Each option may be used once, more than once or not at all.

24. A 37-year-old parous woman with two children is suffering from long-standing heavy menstrual bleeding. She has tried various hormonal and non-hormonal methods in the past including a levonorgestrel-releasing intrauterine system. Her partner had a vasectomy few years ago. She is now seeking a permanent solution to her heavy and painful periods. She is a non-smoker and has recently lost a stone; her current body mass index is 37. Her recent endometrial biopsy is normal and she is up to date with her smears.

25. A 44-year-old woman is known to have heavy menstrual bleeding and uterine fibroids. She has had regular periods while on the combined oral contraceptive pill and tranexamic acid for the last 2 years, but her periods have recently become erratic. She has a 14-year-old child with special needs and being a single parent she finds it difficult to take care of him. Her general practitioner requests a scan which shows three intramural fibroids, the largest measuring 6 cm. Upon examination her uterine size is 15 weeks of pregnancy.

Questions 26 – 27

Options list for Questions 26 – 27

A   Lichen sclerosus
B   Eczema
C   Vulval intraepithelial neoplasia
D   Allergic dermatitis
E   Crohn's disease
F   Vitiligo
G   Psoriasis
H   Genital herpes
I   Squamous cell carcinoma
J   Vulval wart
K   Atrophic vulvovaginitis
L   Lichen planus
M   Vulvodynia

For each patient described below, choose the single most likely diagnosis from the above list of options. Each option may be used once, more than once, or not at all.

26. A 28-year-old woman presents to you complaining of vulval itching. On further inquiry, she claims that she has not been able to have intercourse with her partner lately due to pain. She doesn't give any history of allergies in the past. On examination, there are small fissures in interlabial sulci.

27. A 49-year-old woman presents to you complaining of vulval skin irritation and painful intercourse. On examination you can see that the vulval skin is thickened, erythematous and has areas of brown pigmentation. VIN

Questions 28 – 29

Option list for Questions 28 – 29:

A Ectropion
B Cervical polyp
C Cervical intraepithelial neoplasia
D Carcinoma of the cervix
E Chronic cervicitis
F Human papilloma virus infection

G Actinomycosis
H Nabothian follicle
I Cervical fibroid
J Cervical endometriosis
K Trichomoniasis

For each clinical scenario described below, choose the single most likely diagnosis from the above list of options. Each option may be used once, more than once, or not at all.

28. A 27-year-old woman presents with post-coital bleeding. Upon speculum examination her cervix appears patulous, erythematous and oedematous (**Figure 15.1**).

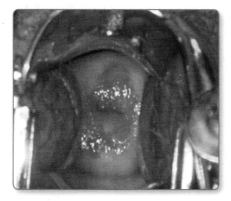

Figure 15.1 Oedematous and erythematous cervix.

29. A 32-year-old woman presents to the clinic complaining of dyspareunia and vaginal spotting for 3–4 months. Bimanual examination is uncomfortable for her and her cervix shows macular lesions with pigmented areas (**Figure 15.2**) on speculum examination.

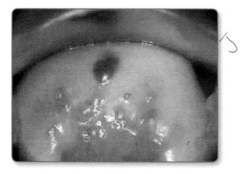

Figure 15.2 Ill-defined macular lesion with pigmented spots.

Questions 30 – 31

Options list for Questions 30 – 31

A   Conservative management
B   Ultrasound-guided aspiration
C   Laparoscopic ovarian cystectomy
D   Laparoscopic oophorectomy
E   Measurement of CA-125
F   Repeat ultrasound

G   Laparoscopic aspiration
H   Measurement of lactate
    dehydrogenase, α-fetoprotein and
    β-hCG levels in the blood
I   Combined oral contraceptive pill
J   Laparotomy

For each case described below, choose the single most likely management option from the above list of options. Each option may be used once, more than once, or not at all.

30. A 26-year-old woman presents at 14 weeks in her first pregnancy, with recurrent lower abdominal pain that suddenly increased yesterday. She has vomited a few times since last night. Clinically she looks to be in pain and is haemodynamically stable; she is tender in the right lower quadrant. Her blood and urine tests are normal. Ultrasound scan shows a right-sided ovarian cyst measuring $8 \times 6 \times 7.2$ cm with internal echoes, alongside a viable intrauterine pregnancy of 14 weeks. Your clinical suspicion is torsion ovarian cyst.

31. A 42-year-old woman presents with abdominal pain. During investigations she is found to have a large left-sided complex ovarian cyst.

Questions 32 – 33

Options list for Questions 32 – 33:

A   Functional
B   Endometrioma
C   Serous cystadenoma
D   Mucinous cystadenoma
E   Dermoid cyst

F   Paratubal cyst
G   Hydrosalpinx
H   Pelvic kidney
I   Germ cell tumour
J   Epithelial carcinoma

For each clinical scenario described below, choose the single most likely diagnosis from the above list of options. Each option may be used once, more than once, or not at all.

32. A 28-year-old woman presents with dull, chronic lower abdominal pain. On a pelvic scan, a large complex unilocular cystic mass is seen in the left adnexa, with thin internal septations. There is no obvious wall thickness or nodularity. On Doppler ultrasonography, no abnormal vascularity is noted within the septations. Her left ovary cannot be seen separate from the mass.

33. A 32-year-old woman is referred from the emergency department for a gynaecological opinion. She has presented with lower abdominal pain and has been seen by surgeons to rule out appendicitis. She is clinically stable with no specific tenderness or guarding. Her white blood cell count and C-reactive protein are slightly raised. Her ultrasound scan shows a structure with a 'cogwheel' appearance in the right adnexa.

Answers: SBAs

1. C Endometrial biopsy

In women aged 45 years or over, endometrial biopsy should be performed in order to exclude endometrial hyperplasia or cancer.

2. C Antifibrinolytic

Tranexamic acid is an antifibrinolytic. It works by preventing blood clots from breaking down too quickly.

Examples of COX inhibitors are celecoxib and acetylsalicylic acid.

An example of a menstrual endometrium stabiliser is ethamsylate.

3. D Smear and HPV testing at a general practice 6 months post LLETZ

In April 2010 the UK National Cervical Cancer Screening Service introduced human papilloma virus (HPV) triage. This meant that women who have had treatment for high-grade disease should now have a cervical smear initially for follow up. If it is abnormal the patient is then seen at the colposcopy clinic. If normal the smear is tested for HPV. If it is HPV-positive the patient is also referred the colposcopy clinic, but if negative the patient goes back to routine recall.

4. E Repeat the pelvic ultrasound and CA-125 in 4 months

Simple, unilateral unilocular cysts less than 5 cm have a very low risk of malignancy (less than 1%) and can be managed conservatively (RCOG green top guideline 34). Given she is asymptomatic and this is an incidental finding, conservative management is reasonable.

5. C Crown-rump length of 8.6 mm with no fetal heart

A missed miscarriage is diagnosed if the crown-rump length is 7.0 mm or more with a transvaginal ultrasound scan and there is no visible heartbeat, or if the mean gestational sac diameter is 25.0 mm or more using a transvaginal ultrasound scan and there is no visible fetal pole.

Except for option C, the other stems do not fit the criteria. These are pregnancies of uncertain viability and the scan needs to be repeated after 1–2 weeks.

6. D Stable patient with β-hCG of 1487 IU/L and minimal free fluid in the pouch of Douglas (POD)

Offer systemic methotrexate as a first-line treatment to women who are able to return for follow-up and who have all of the following: no significant pain, an unruptured ectopic pregnancy with an adnexal mass smaller than 35 mm with no visible heartbeat, a serum β-hCG level less than 1500 IU/L, no intrauterine pregnancy (as confirmed on an ultrasound scan).

Offer surgery where treatment with methotrexate is not acceptable to the woman.

Offer surgery as a first-line treatment to women who are unable to return for follow-up after methotrexate treatment or who have any of the following:

- an ectopic pregnancy and significant pain
- an ectopic pregnancy with an adnexal mass of 35 mm or larger
- an ectopic pregnancy with a fetal heartbeat visible on an ultrasound scan
- an ectopic pregnancy and a serum β-hCG level of 5000 IU/L or more

Offer the choice of either methotrexate or surgical management to women with an ectopic pregnancy who have a serum β-hCG level of at least 1500 IU/L and less than 5000 IU/L, who are able to return for follow-up and who meet all of the following criteria: no significant pain, an unruptured ectopic pregnancy with an adnexal mass smaller than 35 mm with no visible heartbeat and no intrauterine pregnancy (as confirmed on an ultrasound scan).

7. B Hysteroscopic fibroid resection

A levonorgestrel-releasing intrauterine system is not suitable for a grade 0 fibroid. Pregnancy is not advisable after uterine artery embolisation. Gonadotropin-releasing hormone (GnRH) analogues will not cure the problem but provide temporary relief. Hysterectomy is not an option if patient wants to preserve her fertility. Submucous fibroid can affect fertility and its removal offers the best chance to achieve symptomatic relief as well as improve the chances of conception.

8. D Cyclical progestogens

Cyclical mood swings and bloating are likely to be due to increased progesterone in secretory (premenstrual) phase of the cycle. Using cyclical progestogens may therefore worsen the symptoms.

9. E Repeat ultrasound scan

The above scenario suggests that the patient might be having tubal miscarriage or ruptured ectopic pregnancy. Surgical management will be suggested if the patient is unstable which is not given in the scenario. Before deciding on 2nd dose methotrexate, the patient should have an ultrasound scan to check the following: size of ectopic mass change, presence of haemoperitoneum or any abnormal findings that may contradict the use of 2nd methotrexate dose.

10. B Transvaginal scan in 2 weeks

According to NICE guidelines, if there is no visible fetal heartbeat ('uncertain viability') on a transabdominal scan and the fetal pole is not visible, record the mean gestational sac diameter and perform a second scan in a minimum of 14 days before making a diagnosis. For transvaginal scan on first assessment the second scan should be performed a minimum of 7 days after the first scan before making a diagnosis.

11. C Misoprostol 400 µg vaginal

In outpatient management of miscarriage, a 400 µg dose of vaginal misoprostol appears to be as effective at inducing complete miscarriage as an 800 µg dose, and is associated with a reduced rate of fever and rigors, and improved patient satisfaction.

12. D Hysteroscopic resection of polyp under general anaesthetic

Due to the size of the polyp, resection is best done under direct vision.

Answers: EMQs

13. J Pelvic inflammatory disease (PID)

She is less than 25 and has had a number of sexual partners. The history is not suggestive of endometriosis and PID seems more likely.

14. D Endosalpingiosis

Endosalpingiosis is a condition where cells from the fallopian tube are found in ectopic locations. It is uncertain what clinical significance this condition has.

15. F Hydrosalpinx

The description is that of a hydrosalpinx and this fits best with her history, in particular the previous sexually transmitted infection.

16. A Adenomyosis

The symptoms are suggestive of adenomyosis. Heavy bleeding can be associated with endometriosis but the tender enlargement of the uterus suggests adenomyosis. Fibroids do not tend to be tender upon palpation.

17. M None of the above

The diagnosis is not clear in this situation. Pelvic inflammatory disease seems unlikely and it is not long enough in duration to be classed as chronic pelvic pain.

18. B Endometrioma

The history is highly suggestive of endometriosis and the scan findings are characteristic. If scan findings were ambiguous a MRI would be warranted. CA-125 can be substantially raised in endometriosis.

19. M Tubo-ovarian abscess

The history is suggestive of pelvic inflammatory disease (PID) and the scan findings are suggestive of PID with sequlae of tuboovarian abscess.

20. E Mature cystic ovarian teratoma

These are one of the most common reasons for ovarian cystectomies in pre-menopausal woman, and the scan findings are characteristic.

21. D Haemorrhagic cyst

The history is highly suggestive of an acute event such as bleeding or torsion. The pelvic scan findings point more towards a haemorrhagic cyst.

22. B Hysterectomy

Hysterectomy seems to be the appropriate option in this situation because of increased bleeding and pressure symptoms. This seems to be the correct choice for her age and parity. Hysterectomy remains a definitive and permanent treatment of fibroids that shows highest satisfaction rates regarding heavy bleeding and pressure symptoms. However, hysterectomy is a major surgical procedure associated with longer hospital stay and increased time off from work.

23. I Tranexamic acid

Tranexemic acid is an antifibrinolytic drug and is frequently used in the treatment of heavy menstrual bleeding. Evidence supports, that it may reduce menorrhagia as well as blood loss at the time of myomectomy. This is a correct choice for her as compared to myomectomy keeping in view her age approaching menopause. Also, as there has been no significant change in the size of fibroids, her symptoms could be attributed to climacteric. A levonorgestrel-releasing intrauterine system is not an option here due to the size of the fibroid.

24. E Endometrial ablation

Treatment of heavy menstrual bleeding with obesity is challenging. Raised body mass index (BMI) is associated with poor efficacy of hormonal contraception. Hysterectomy will have additional complications in the presence of a raised BMI. She should be counselled about ablation which destroys the endometrial lining and avoids risks of GA and a major surgery like hysterectomy.

25. G Hysterectomy

Considering her age and social circumstances, conservation of her uterus will not confer any benefit. Hysterectomy is the most appropriate choice of treatment. Abdominal hysterectomy is indicated with a uterine size of 15 weeks. A subtotal abdominal hysterectomy may be performed according to patient preference or if surgery is technically difficult. In young patients with menorrhagia, the ovaries are usually conserved but a bilateral salpingo-oophorectomy may be carried out after detailed discussion with the patient, with particular attention to family history. Women should be counselled about 1:72 lifelong risk of developing ovarian cancer if the ovaries have been retained at hysterectomy.

26. B Eczema

Vulval fissuring is usually due to dermatitis or eczema. In the absence of history of allergies, eczema is a more likely diagnosis.

27. C Vulval intraepithelial neoplasia (VIN)

VIN can be asymptomatic, but can also present with pain, discomfort, irritation or vulval ulceration. On examination, vulva may appear glazed, erythematous, thickened, macerated skin or brown pigmentation. There can be a combination of all these on appearance. Untreated VIN may proceed to invasive cancer.

28. E Chronic cervicitis

Chronic cervicitis is caused by infections like sexually-transmitted infections; allergies, e.g. spermicides; irritation, e.g. arising from the use of a diaphragm; hormonal treatment; cancer or cancer treatment.

29. J Cervical endometriosis

The cervix is a rare location for endometriosis. When present, this condition is associated with perimenstrual spotting and contact bleeding, although most of the patients may be asysmptomatic. The appearance of the lesions may vary just like intraperitoneal endometriotic lesions.

30. C Laparoscopic ovarian cystectomy

A laparoscopy is the most suitable option in clinically stable patients. Oophorectomy is performed if the ovarian tissue is no more viable or if the cyst occupies most of the ovarian surface. This decision is best made when ovary is seen under direct vision. As this scenario doesn't give any details about it, laparoscopic cystectomy is the most appropriate choice of managements from the provided list.

31. J Measurement of lactate dehydrogenase, α-fetoprotein and β-hCG levels in the blood

Although laparoscopic ovarian cystectomy has become the standard approach, laparotomy still remains an alternative approach. Indications for laparotomy are large, complex cysts and cysts that are suspected to be malignant.

32. C Serous cystadenoma

Cystadenomas are the most common benign tumours and are typically large tumours. The type depends on their inner epithelium. Inner epithelium can secrete either serous or mucinous fluid. Serous cystadenomas are usually unilocular while mucinous are bilocular.

33. G Hydrosalpinx

A 'cogwheel' sign in pelvic imaging is typical seen in tubal inflammation in pelvic inflammatory disease with hydrosalpinx or pyosalpinx. This is due to the thickening of loops of fallopian tube on cross sectional image. There are infolding projections (which sometimes look like nodules) into the lumen of the fallopian tube, giving the appearance of a cogwheel.

Chapter 16

Contraception

Questions: MCQs

Answer each stem 'True' or 'False'.

1. The following drugs reduce the effectiveness of the combined oral contraceptive pill:
    - A   Azithromycin
    - B   Lamotrigine
    - C   Penicillin
    - D   Phenytoin
    - E   Barbiturates

Questions: SBAs

For the following question, select the single best answer from the five options listed.

2. A 33-year-old woman with a copper intrauterine contraceptive device develops lower abdominal pain and abnormal vaginal discharge with a temperature of 38°C. The patient had sexual intercourse 4 days before the onset of symptoms. She does not want to become pregnant.

    What is the next step in this patient's management?

    - A   Perform an ultrasound scan to confirm the presence of the intrauterine contraceptive device (IUCD)
    - B   Remove the IUCD
    - C   Remove the IUCD and offer the combined oral contraceptive pill
    - D   Start antibiotics for pelvic inflammatory disease and review in 72 hours
    - E   Take swabs for infection screening

Answers: MCQs

1. A False

    B False

    C False

    D True

    E True

    The latest evidence suggests that antibiotic treatment does not reduce the efficacy of the combined oral contraceptive pill (COCP) with the exception of when the patient is suffering from vomiting or diarrhoea. Generally, the efficacy of the combined oral contraceptive is not affected by lamotrigine, but the dose of lamotrigine needs to be adjusted. Phenytoin, carbamazepine and barbiturates are enzyme inducers which increase the metabolism of oestrogens and progestogens in the liver. This may in turn reduce the contraceptive efficacy of the COCP.

Answers: SBAs

2. D Start antibiotics for pelvic inflammatory disease and review in 72 hours

Removing the intrauterine contraceptive device (IUCD) is not going to treat infection, and if a woman diagnosed with pelvic infection wishes to continue to use an IUCD there is no need for routine removal, therefore appropriate antibiotic treatment can be initiated. The British Association for Sexual Health and HIV guidance suggests that there may be better short-term clinical outcomes from IUD removal, and that the decision to remove an IUD in women with PID needs to be balanced against the risk of pregnancy in those women who may have had sex in the preceding 7 days. Follow-up of women with a pelvic infection is advised 72 hours after starting treatment. Further follow-up may be warranted 2–4 weeks after treatment.

Chapter 17

Menopause

Questions: MCQs

Answer each stem 'True' or 'False'.

1. **Regarding premature ovarian failure:**
   - x A   It is responsible for 40% of cases of secondary amenorrhoea
   - B   It affects 0.1% of women under the age of 30 years
   - C   It is defined as 12 months of amenorrhoea before the age of 40 years
   - D   A single measurement of follicle-stimulating hormone > 30 IU/L is diagnostic
   - E   Once it has been confirmed, contraception is no longer needed

2. **When considering the menopausal patient, obesity has a negative impact on the pathogenesis of these conditions:**
   - A   Breast cancer
   - B   Endometrial cancer
   - C   Cardiovascular disease
   - D   Osteoporosis
   - E   Urogenital dysfunction

3. **Menopausal symptoms:**
   - A   Occur in 50% of women   85%
   - B   Vasomotor symptoms are the most common symptom in Caucasian women
   - C   Are more likely to be experienced by women with higher anxiety levels and higher perceived levels of stress
   - D   Last for a median length of time of 2 years   4/.
   - E   May persist for 15 years after menopause in 1% of the population   6/.

4. **A 48-year-old woman with a body mass index of 24 is perimenopausal with mild vasomotor symptoms.**

   Which of these are contraceptive options for this patient?
   - A   Copper intrauterine device
   - B   Depo progesterone
   - C   Combined oral contraceptive pill
   - D   Oestrogen-only hormone replacement therapy with uterine levonorgestrel intrauterine system
   - E   Sequential combined hormone replacement therapy

5. **The following are absolute contraindications to using hormone replacement therapy:**
   A   Active liver disease
   B   Family history of breast cancer
   C   Treatment for oestrogen receptor positive breast cancer 2 years ago
   D   Untreated endometrial hyperplasia
   E   Venous thromboembolism in a first degree relative who broke their ankle at 55 years of age

6. **The following are appropriate management options for osteoporosis prevention:**
   A   1–2 mg of ostradiol daily
   B   0.25–0.50 μg oestradiol patch daily
   C   300–625 mg conjugated equine oestrogen daily
   D   Bisphosphonates
   E   Calcium and vitamin D supplements

Questions: SBAs

For each question, select the single best answer from the five options listed.

7. Which clinical feature is diagnostic of the menopause?

    A   Amenorrhoea for longer than 12 months after the age of 45 years
    B   Follicle stimulating hormone level of > 30 IU/L
    C   Development of vasomotor symptoms
    D   Menstrual changes after the age of 52 years
    E   Sexual dysfunction and reduced libido after the age of 52 years

8. Which of the following conditions is not associated with an early menopause?

    A   Cardiovascular disease
    B   Osteoporosis
    C   Endometrial cancer
    D   Sexual dysfunction
    E   Subfertility

9. Which enzyme is responsible for the peripheral conversion of androgens to oestradiol in the menopausal patient?

    A   P450 aromatase
    B 5α reductase
    C 17α-hydroxylase
    D   17–20 desmolase
    E 17-β hydroxysteroid dehydrogenase

10. A 48-year-old patient with a body mass index of 24 is referred to the gynaecology department because her periods have become more unpredictable and are sometimes heavier than she is used to. Her cycle is now 4–8/28–38. Her last period, which lasted for 8 days and was associated with clots, was 3 weeks ago. Her follicle stimulating hormone level is 12 IU/L.

    What STRAW +10 criteria best fit her current menopausal status?

    A   –5
    B   –4
    C   –3b
    D   –2
    E   –1

11. A 48-year-old patient with a body mass index of 28 is referred to the gynaecology department because she is experiencing vasomotor symptoms. Her last period was 3 months ago and her general practitioner was uncertain whether cyclical hormone replacement therapy or the combined oral contraceptive pill would be most appropriate.

What STRAW +10 criteria best fit her current menopausal status?

    A −4
    B −3b
    C −2
    D −1
    E +1

Questions: EMQs

Questions 12 – 16

Option list for Questions 12 – 16:

A   Addison's disease
B   Chemotherapy
C   Diabetes mellitus
D   Down's syndrome (trisomy 21)
E   Fragile X syndrome
F   Galactosaemia
G   17–20 desmolase deficiency
H   17α-hydroxylase deficiency
I   Hypothyroidism
J   Hysterectomy
K   Idiopathic
L   Inhibin B mutation
M   Mumps
N   Smoking
O   Tuberculosis
P   Turner's syndrome

For each of the following cases, select the single most appropriate cause for premature ovarian failure. Each option may be used once, more than once or not at all.

12. A 35-year-old women presents to her general practitioner with a 14-month history of amenorrhoea. She has an follicle-stimulating hormone level of 42 IU/L.

13. A 29-year-old woman attends the antenatal clinic with her partner to receive the results of her recent amniocentesis. She has attended an appointment with her general practitioner as she is very confused about what she was told. She remembers being told that the baby's genetic material is not completely normal and that the condition will cause delayed puberty, menstrual problems and an early menopause.

14. A 40-year-old woman presents to her general practitioner with a 15-month history of amenorrhoea. She has an follicle-stimulating hormone level of 50 IU/L. She is otherwise well. She smokes 10 cigarettes per day. Her mother went through the menopause at 52 years of age. Her sister is also a smoker and has a normal menstrual pattern.

15. A 34-year-old women presents to her general practitioner with a 7-month history of amenorrhoea. She has an follicle-stimulating hormone level of 45 IU/L. Over the last 9 months she has been feeling increasingly tired and low in mood. She feels the cold much more than she used to and her hair has thinned.

16. A 17-year-old girl presents to the gynaecologist with delayed puberty and primary amenorrhoea. As part of the investigations she is noted to have hypertension and hypokalaemia.

Questions 17 – 21

Option list for questions 17 – 21

A Clonidine
B Combined oral contraceptive pill
C Fluoxetine
D Gabapentin
E Oestrogen and progesterone hormone replacement therapy (continuous)
F Oestrogen and progesterone hormone replacement therapy (cyclical)
G Oestrogen-only hormone replacement therapy
H Oestrogen replacement (oral or patches) + levonorgestrel intrauterine system

I Phyto-oestrogens
J Tibolone
K Testosterone replacement
L Topical hormone replacement therapy patches
M Vaginal oestrogen replacement
N Vaginal lubricants and moisturisers, e.g. Replens, Silc
O Venlafaxine
P None of the above

For each of the following cases, select the single most appropriate management option. Each option may be used once, more than once or not at all.

17. A 40-year-old woman with a body mass index of 28 has undergone a bilateral salpingo-oophorectomy for endometriosis. She has no significant past medical history but has a family history of breast cancer (her mother was diagnosed at 65 years old).

18. A 53-year-old woman with a body mass index of 27 has debilitating vasomotor symptoms. Her last menstrual period was 18 months ago. She has type 1 diabetes mellitus. She has been counselled about the risks of HRT and accepts them.

19. A 53-year-old woman with a body mass index of 35 has debilitating vasomotor symptoms. Her last menstrual period was 18 months ago. She has type 2 diabetes mellitus. She has been counselled about the risks of HRT and accepts them.

20. A 48-year-old woman with a body mass index of 24 has had symptoms of night sweats and poor sleep for 6 months. She is oligomenorrhoeic and her last menstrual period was 4 months ago. Her partner has had a vasectomy.

21. A 47-year-old woman with a body mass index of 30 has minimal menopausal symptoms. She is oligomenorrhoeic and her last menstrual period was 6 months ago. She had some low mood symptoms following breakdown of her marriage 1 year ago, but these are much improved now she has started a new sexual relationship. She does not like the idea of an intrauterine device and her partner does not like condoms.

Question 22 – 26

Option list for Questions 22 – 26:

A   Clonidine
B   Combined oral contraceptive pill
C   Fluoxetine
D   Gabapentin
E   Oestrogen and progesterone hormone replacement therapy (continuous)
F   Oestrogen and progesterone hormone replacement therapy (cyclical)
G   Oestrogen-only hormone replacement therapy
H   Oestrogen replacement (oral or patches) + levonorgestrel intrauterine system

I   Phyto-oestrogens
J   Tibolone
K   Testosterone replacement
L   Topical hormone replacement therapy patches
M   Vaginal oestrogen replacement
N   Vaginal lubricants and moisturisers, e.g. Replens, Silc
O   Venlafaxine
P   None of the above

For each of the following cases, select the single most appropriate management option. Each option may be used once, more than once or not at all.

22. A 60-year-old woman with a body mass index of 22 attends her general practice to discuss symptoms of vaginal dryness and soreness, particularly noticeable after intercourse. Her last menstrual period was 8 years ago. She has read about HRT and is concerned about taking it as she is currently on two different antihypertensive medications.

23. A 45-year-old woman with a body mass index of 29 has had a mastectomy and chemotherapy for oestrogen receptor positive breast cancer. She has been ammenorrhoeic for the last 2 years. She has severe hot flushes and night sweats.

24. A 43-year-old woman with a body mass index of 28 has had a hysterectomy and bilateral salpingo-oophorectomy for fibroids and persistent ovarian cysts. She has no significant past medical history but has a family history of breast cancer (her mother was diagnosed at 65 years old).

25. A 48-year-old woman with a body mass index of 27 has heavy irregular periods. She is also experiencing severe vasomotor symptoms. Her last menstrual period was 2 months ago. Her copper intrauterine contraceptive device is due to be changed this month.

26. A 55-year-old woman with a body mass index of 39 complains of 2 months of vaginal dryness, difficulty with intercourse and mild cystitis symptoms following intercourse. She had a mastectomy and chemotherapy for oestrogen receptor positive breast cancer 8 years ago. She has been menopausal since her treatment.

Question 27 – 31

Option list for Questions 27 – 31

A   Clonidine
B   COCP
C   Fluoxetine
D   Gabapentin
E   Oestrogen and progesterone hormone replacement therapy (continuous)
F   Oestrogen and progesterone hormone replacement therapy (cyclical)
G   Oestrogen-only hormone replacement therapy
H   Oestrogen replacement (oral or patches) + levonorgestrel intrauterine system

I   Phyto-oestrogens
J   Tibolone
K   Testosterone replacement
L   Topical hormone replacement therapy patches
M   Vaginal oestrogen replacement
N   Vaginal lubricants and moisturisers
O   Venlafaxine
P   None of the above

For each of the following cases, select the single most appropriate management option. Each option may be used once, more than once or not at all.

27. A 53-year-old woman with a body mass index of 27 has moderate vasomotor symptoms and a significant reduction in her libido. She is in a relationship with a supportive partner but is finding her symptoms frustrating. She has been advised by her general practitioner not to use hormone replacement therapy as her mother developed deep venous thrombosis at the age of 60 years after breaking her ankle. Her last menstrual period was 2 years ago.

28. A 53-year-old woman with a body mass index of 27 has moderate vasomotor symptoms and a significant reduction in her libido. She is in a good relationship with a supportive partner. She has been on continuous combined hormone replacement therapy for 6 months and her vasomotor symptoms have resolved. Unfortunately there has been no change in her libido and she is finding it is putting a strain on her relationship.

29. A 54-year-old woman with a body mass index of 28 has debilitating vasomotor symptoms. She had a pulmonary embolism 3 months after starting the combined oral contraceptive pill at the age of 22 years. She is otherwise quite fit and well but also has a family history of deep vein thrombosis.

30. A 51-year-old woman with a body mass index of 24 has moderate vasomotor symptoms. She does not want to take anything 'unnatural' or to 'poison her body with any drugs'. She has come to discuss her options for managing menopause.

31. A 53-year-old woman with a body mass index of 25 has moderate vasomotor symptoms. Her past medical history includes a mastectomy and chemotherapy for oestrogen receptor positive breast cancer 2 years ago. She is currently taking tamoxifen. She has come to discuss her options for managing menopause. She does not want to take anything 'unnatural' or 'poison her body with any drugs'.

Answers: MCQs

1. A False

    B True

    C True

    D False

    E False

    Premature ovarian failure (POF) is responsible for 4–18% of secondary and 10–28% of primary amenorrhoea. Two measurements > 30 IU/L 6 weeks apart or a single measurement > 40 IU/L. 1% of the patient's with POF have spontaneous ovulation and so pregnancy is possible.

2. A True

    B True

    C True

    D False

    E True

    Obesity has a negative impact on most health conditions but the increased peripheral conversion of androgens to oestradiol makes osteoporosis less likely in this population. The risk of osteoarthritis is worsened by obesity. Osteoporosis is associated with a low body mass index.

3. A False

    B True

    C True

    D False

    E False

    Menopausal symptoms occur in 85% of women. With relatively similar endocrine changes, symptom reporting should be generalised, yet more women in Western countries report vasomotor symptoms (hot flushes and night sweats) compared with women in Asian countries. The median duration of symptom is 4 years (1–6 years). In 10% of the population, vasomotor symptoms persist some 15 years after menopause. Anxiety can strike at any time during woman's life, but stages of hormonal fluctuations can trigger anxiety episodes, therefore anxiety is not uncommon during menopause.

4. A True

    B True

    C True

D True

E False

The copper intrauterine device and depot medroxyprogesterone acetate contraceptive injection can be used for contraception through the menopause and beyond 50. Current guidance is that the combined oral contraceptive pill can be used until the age of 50 years. Although oestrogen replacement with a levonorgestrel intrauterine system is often suggested for management of menopausal symptoms it would also provide contraception. Combined hormone replacement therapy preparations, either sequential or continuous do not provide contraception and patients should be made aware of this as pregnancy is still possible in these patients.

5. A True

B False

C True

D True

E False

A family history of breast cancer is a relative contraindication and should be explored as part of the counselling process for patients wanting to take HRT.

This venous thromboembolism (VTE) has occurred following trauma, after the age of 50 years, and is not oestrogen dependent so does not influence the patient's individual risk of VTE.

6. A True

B False

C False

D True

E True

The basis of this question is an understanding of the type of prevention options available to patients and knowledge of the minimum dose of oestrogen replacement to provide bone protection.

Answers: SBAs

7. A Amenorrhoea for longer than 12 months after the age of 45 years

The menopause is recognised to have occurred after 12 months of amenorrhoea for which no other obvious pathological or physiological cause is present.

8. C Endometrial cancer

There is an association between delayed menopause and a raised risk of oestrogen-dependent cancers such as endometrial cancer and breast cancer.

9. A P450 aromatase

P450 aromatase is responsible for the conversion.

10. D −2

She is in the early perimenopause with variable periods- increased bleeding time and ≥ 7-day difference between one cycle and the next. Follicle-stimulating hormone test results are variable at this time, which is why they can be unreliable for making a diagnosis. These features are consistent with STRAW -2.

Chronological age is an unreliable indicator of menopause so an internationally recognised standard for characterising and classifying reproductive ageing was developed in 2001 at the Stages of Reproductive Ageing Workshop (STRAW). This defined five stages prior to the final menstrual period (FMP) and 2 afterwards. It was then refined in 2011 to create STRAW +10 with subdivisions of the −3 and +1 stage.

11. D −1

Chronological age is unreliable as an indicator of menopause so an internationally recognised standard for characterising and classifying reproductive aging was developed in 2001 at the Stages of Reproductive Ageing Workshop (STRAW). This defined five stages prior to the final menstrual period and two afterwards. It was then refined in 2011 to create STRAW +10 with subdivisions of the -3 and +1 stage. All the stages are shown in O'Niel et al., 2014.

Answers: EMQs

12. K Idiopathic

No cause is found in the majority of cases.

13. P Turner's syndrome

Turner's syndrome is most likely from the description given. Down's syndrome can be associated with premature ovarian insufficiency but not delayed puberty.

14. K Idiopathic

Although smoking is associated with a natural menopause happening 1–2 years earlier than expected this seems unlikely to be the cause in this situation. Again an idiopathic cause is most likely.

15. I Hypothyroidism

This is a classic description of hypothyroidism. Autoimmune hypothyroidism is associated with premature ovarian insufficiency in 25% of cases.

16. H 17α-hydroxylase deficiency

The increased mineralocorticoid production leading to hypertension and hypokalaemia makes this enzyme deficiency the most likely cause.

17. J Tibolone

Tibolone is the most appropriate drug for use in hormone replacement therapy for endometriosis. Her risk of breast cancer is no different to the background population and the risk of osteoporosis and cardiovascular disease outweigh her breast cancer risk until she is 50 years of age.

18. E Oestrogen and progesterone hormone replacement therapy (continuous)

Continuous combined HRT is appropriate as her last menstrual period was > 12 months ago.

19. L Topical hormone replacement therapy patches

Her body mass index puts her at greater risk of venous thromboembolism (VTE) and current guidelines recommend topical hormone replacement therapy (HRT) to avoid the impact of HRT on the liver and so the risk of VTE.

20. F Oestrogen and progesterone hormone replacement therapy (cyclical)

Cyclical combined hormone replacement therapy is appropriate. She would need counselling about contraception in this situation had her partner not had a vasectomy. If contraception was needed, oestrogen replacement (oral or patches) + levonorgestrel- intrauterine system would have been a more appropriate management option.

21. B Combined oral contraceptive pill

Her symptoms are minimal and she needs contraception. A trial of the combined oral contraceptive pill would be reasonable to see what effect this has on her symptoms. Using progesterone-only contraception would not address her menopausal symptoms.

22. M Vaginal oestrogen replacement

Adequate vaginal oestrogenisation may improve all of these symptoms. There is no clinically significant absorption of oestrogen so this therapy would have no influence on her stroke risk.

23. O Venlafaxine

Oestrogen replacement is not appropriate. A trial of serotonin–norepinephrine reuptake inhibitor would be an option.

24. G Oestrogen-only hormone replacement therapy

She is young and would benefit from oestrogen replacement. She does not require progesterone. Her family history does not influence her risk.

25. H Oestrogen replacement (oral or patches) + levonorgestrel intrauterine system

Her copper IUD might be contributing to her symptoms and she would benefit from oestrogen replacement.

26. O Vaginal lubricants and moisturisers

There is no clinically significant absorption of vaginal oestrogen replacement but there is no evidence to support its use in oestrogen receptor positive breast cancer. It may be an option but should not be used as a first line treatment and should be discussed with oncology before prescribing. Her option for first line treatment is vaginal lubricants and moisturisers.

27. E Oestrogen and progesterone hormone replacement therapy (continuous)

She is symptomatic and would benefit from hormone replacement therapy (oestrogen) would benefit both vasomotor and libido symptoms. Oestrogen and progesterone replacement is necessary as there is nothing to suggest she has had a hysterectomy. The family history does not put her at a significantly increased risk but the risks of hormone replacement therapy would need to be discussed.

28. H Oestrogen replacement (oral or patches) + levonorgestrel intrauterine system

Once appropriate oestrogen replacement has occurred and if symptoms of libido remain an issue a trial of testosterone replacement can be considered.

29. P None of the above

She has a high risk of venous thromboembolism so a referral to haematology for a thrombophilia screen would be appropriate prior to any decision on hormone replacement therapy.

30. I Phyto-oestrogens

Phyto-oestrogens are naturally occurring oestrogens that some patients prefer. They should be aware that these are associated with the same risks as human oestrogens, and should therefore be avoided if an oncologist advises a patient to avoid oestrogen replacement.

31. O Venlafaxine

Venlafaxine reduces the severity of hot flushes in menopausal women. The exact mechanism of action is not known.

Chapter 18

Surgical interventions

Questions: MCQs

Answer each stem 'True' or 'False'.

1. The following are recognised risks at the time of the insertion of a trocar:
   - A   Risk of bowel damage is about 1%   4/10 000
   - B   Risk of damage to major blood vessels is 1 in 500 cases   2/10 000
   - C   The risk of major blood vessel injury can be minimised by using direct entry technique with blunt vista ports
   - D   Hasson direct trocar insertion is safer compared with a Veress needle introduction technique
   - E   Open entry technique is recommended for very thin patients

Questions: SBAs

For each question, select the single best answer from the five options listed.

2. You are about to consent a patient for diagnostic laparoscopy. Her body mass index is 22 kg/m2 and has no history of previous abdominal surgery. The patient wishes to know about the serious complications associated with laparoscopy. She is anxious as her friend required an open operation to repair her bowel following a laparoscopic sterilisation. In counselling her you should include:

    A   A serious complication like a bowel injury is recognised at the time of surgery and dealt with immediately

    B   Wound gaping and infection can lead to serious intraperitoneal infection

    C   Serious complications associated with bowel injury during entry can be avoided if the open technique entry is used

    D   The overall risk of serious complications is low: approximately 2 in 1000 women

    E   A serious complication like a blood vessel injury in her case is reduced as easy entry to the abdominal cavity is anticipated

3. You are asked to include the risk of 'return to theatre' as one of the complications following hysterectomy in patient information leaflet and consent form.

    Which one of the following figures should be quoted in the consent form?

    A   2 in 100

    B   15 in 1000

    C   7 in 1000

    D   5 in 10000

    E   1 in 100 following hysterectomy for malignant disease

4. Which of the following operations is associated with the highest incidence of postoperative fever?

    A   Vaginal hysterectomy

    B   Laparoscopic hysterectomy

    C   Abdominal hysterectomy

    D   Sacrospinous colpopexy

    E   Anterior and posterior repair

5. Of the following operations which one is associated with the highest incidence of vault haematoma?

    A   Laparoscopic hysterectomy

    B   Abdominal hysterectomy

    C   Abdominal myomectomy

    D   Vaginal hysterectomy

    E   Robotic hysterectomy

6. What is the risk of death as a result of complications during a laparoscopic procedure?

    A 5–8 in 10000
    B 2 in 100000
    C 3–8 in 100000
    D 1 in 1000
    E 1 in 10000

7. Your consultant has asked you to identify and name the blood vessel in the abdominal wall which is most likely to be injured during lateral port insertion during laparoscopy.

    A Superficial epigastric
    B Inferior epigastric
    C Superficial circumflex iliac
    D External iliac
    E Superior epigastric

8. What should be the intra-abdominal pressure (IAP) during laparoscopy?

    A IAP 20–25 mmHg before the insertion of the primary trocar
    B IAP 10–12 mmHg before the insertion of secondary trocars
    C IAP 10–12 mmHg before the insertion of the primary trocar
    D IAP 25 mmHg during the laparoscopic procedure after the insertion of trocars
    E IAP 15 mmHg before the insertion of the primary trocar

9. Hassan's entry technique or Palmer's point is not recommended in which of the following?

    A Very thin women
    B Morbidly obese women
    C Previous vertical abdominal incision
    D Previous caesarean section
    E Previous multiple laparoscopies

10. The highest risk of vascular injury during laparoscopy is in which of the following?

    A Multiparous thin women
    B Thin nulliparous women
    C Morbidly obese and nulliparous women
    D Patients with multiple laparotomies
    E Morbidly obese and multiparous women

11. One of the following statements is true about hysteroscopic distension media?

    A Normal saline causes more vasovagal symptoms than CO_2
    B Normal saline has better image quality than CO_2
    C CO_2 use leads to a quicker procedure
    D CO_2 has better image quality than normal saline
    E Normal saline is usually used for monopolar diathermy

12. A thin 51-year-old woman undergoes total laparoscopic hysterectomy for dysfunctional uterine bleeding. The procedure is uneventful with minimal blood loss. The patient is fully mobile and is discharged home the next day.

How long will you advice postoperative thromboprophylaxis for this patient?

   A   14 days
   B   7 days
   C   28 days
   D   42 days
   E   None

13. An 18-year-old woman, who is 5 weeks pregnant, complains of severe lower abdominal pain and vaginal bleeding. On examination, she is noted to have a blood pressure of 80/60 mmHg and heart rate of 110 bpm. The serum β-hCG level is 600 mIU/mL and the transvaginal ultrasound shows no intrauterine pregnancy and no obvious adnexal masses. There is some anechoic free fluid in the pouch of Douglas.

Which of the following is the best management for this patient?

   A   Measure the patient's serum progesterone level
   B   Laparoscopy + salpingectomy
   C   Laparotomy + salpingectomy
   D   Intramuscular methotrexate at a dose of 50 mg/m^2
   E   Repeat serum β-hCG in 48 hours

Questions: EMQs

Questions 14 – 18

Option list for Questions 14 – 18:

A	Bladder perforation	G	Post-operative pain
B	Bowel injury	H	Surgical emphysema
C	Bradycardia	I	Thromboembolism
D	Inferior epigastric vessel injury	J	Unrecognised visceral injury
E	Omental injury	K	Uterine perforation
F	Port site hernia	L	Vessel injury

For each of the following cases, select the single most likely complication from the list above. Each option may be used once, more than once or not at all.

14. A 30-year-old woman with a body mass index of 32 was admitted for laparoscopic management of her endometriosis. She had Grade III endometriosis requiring extensive peritoneal excision from the left pelvic side wall and right para-rectal space. She has been readmitted 48 hours after surgery with shortness of breath and a tachycardia.

15. A 24-year-old woman with a body mass index of 18 was admitted to the day surgery unit for a diagnostic laparoscopy to investigate pelvic pain. She has no significant past medical history. After the primary laparoscopic port was placed, the operating surgeon was explaining to a medical student the vasculature of the anterior abdominal wall. The anaesthetist urgently asked for the abdomen to be deflated.

16. A 40-year-old woman with a body mass index of 28 was admitted for laparoscopic division of adhesions following her caesarean section. In view of her previous surgery an open entry technique was used at the umbilicus. During entry of the abdominal cavity yellow, frothy fluid was noted and the operative surgery requested assistance from a senior colleague.

17. A 28-year-old woman with a body mass index of 26 was admitted for hysteroscopy, dilatation and curettage and diagnostic laparoscopy. Laparoscopic entry is uneventful but 150 mL of fresh blood is noted in the pelvis. On closer inspection there is a bleeding point on the uterine fundus.

18. A 25-year-old woman with a body mass index of 29 is admitted to the day surgery unit for a diagnostic laparoscopy and dye test. After insertion of the lateral operative port in the left iliac fossa, brisk bleeding is noted.

Questions 19 – 20

Options list for Questions 19 – 20:

A	Laparoscopic salpingectomy	D	Immediate laparotomy
B	Laparoscopic salpingotomy	E	Conservative management
C	Intramuscular methotrexate	F	Cornual resection

G Hysterectomy	injection of methotrexate in the sac
H Hysteroscopic aspiration	**J** Suction evacuation
I Ultrasound guided aspiration +	

For each case described below, choose the single most likely management option from the above list of options. Each option may be used once, more than once, or not at all.

19. A 23-year-old primigravid woman presents after 7 weeks of amenorrhea with right-sided lower abdominal pain and bleeding per vagina. Her β-hCG is 2850 IU/L. A transvaginal scan shows a small sac like structure in-utero and a heterogeneous, doughnut-like structure in the right adnexa measuring 1.8 × 2 cm. There is no evidence of any cardiac activity within this mass, and no evidence of fluid in pouch of Douglas. The woman is not very keen on a repeat β-hCG and wants treatment straight away. You suspect a right-sided ectopic pregnancy.

20. A 27-year-old woman presents soon after missing her periods. She gives a history of previous two ectopic pregnancies, first treated with right salpingostomy with a subsequent ectopic on the left side treated by methotrexate. She is very worried about the status of her present pregnancy and would prefer an early intervention if this is another ectopic pregnancy. She does feel slight left-sided lower abdominal discomfort, but has no bleeding per vaginum. Clinically, she is haemodynamically stable and there is no tenderness or guarding in her abdomen. Her β-hCG measured today is 1050 IU/L and a transvaginal scan shows a suspicious area near the left cornua, with no clear evidence of an intra-or extra-uterine pregnancy.

Questions 21 – 22

Options list for Questions 21 – 22:

A CT Urogram		**F** Laparotomy
B X-ray abdomen		**G** Ultrasound
C Full blood count		**H** MRI
D Urea and electrolytes		**I** Bladder scan
E Laparoscopy		**J** Urinary self-retaining catheter

For each case described below, choose the single most likely initial treatment option from the above list of options. Each option may be used once, more than once, or not at all.

21. A 43-year-old woman has had a total abdominal hysterectomy because she had multiple uterine fibroids. The procedure was technically difficult due a distorted anatomy. She presented 5 days later with abdominal pain and raised temperature. She complains of burning micturition. On examination, her wound looks slightly inflamed and there is tenderness, fullness and guarding in the right lower abdomen.

22. A 45-year-old woman undergoes a total laparoscopic hysterectomy with bilateral salpingo-oophorectomy. The right ureter is noted to be hitched up and was carefully dissected at the time of hysterectomy. Postoperatively, she complains of abdominal pain mainly on the right and in her right flank.

Questions 23 – 24

Options list for Questions 23 – 24:

A	Bleeding	G	Hernia
B	Infection	H	Bowel injury
C	Haematoma	I	Scar dehiscence
D	Bladder injury	J	Pulmonary oedema
E	Ureteric injury	K	Uterine perforation
F	Pulmonary embolism		

For each patient described below, choose the single most likely diagnosis from the above list of options. Each option may be used once, more than once, or not at all.

23. A 32-year-old woman has undergone laparoscopy for endometriosis. She was found to have dense adhesions along with multiple endometriotic lesions. Lesions were resected and adhesiolysis performed using sharp and thermal dissection. She was discharged from hospital the next day following a smooth recovery. She presented to emergency 2 days later complaining of severe generalised abdominal pain, vomiting, fever and she looks generally unwell.

24. A 32-year-old nulliparous woman is undergoing a hysteroscopic resection of a partial uterine septum as a part of subfertility treatment. Examination under anaesthesia reveals a normal size, irregular shaped retroverted uterus. There was some resistance at the initial access through the cervix, but the resection was performed under direct vision and a good intrauterine view was obtained. Some time after the resection is started, the anaesthetist tells you that the patient is hypotensive.

Questions 25 – 26

Options list for Questions 25 – 26:

A	Uterine perforation, 1–2 in every 100	F	Scar dehiscence 2.4 in 1000
B	Bowel injury, undiagnosed intraoperatively	G	Bladder injury, very rare
		H	Risk of serious complications of 2 in 1000
C	Ureteric injury		
D	Bleeding requiring transfusion	I	Risk of death (3–8 in 100,000)
E	Failure to enter in the abdominal cavity	J	Failure rate of 1 in 200

For each procedure described below, from the above list of options choose the single most relevant complication that must be discussed with the patient while taking consent prior to surgery. Each option may be used once, more than once, or not at all.

25. A 45-year-old woman presents with abnormal uterine bleeding and is undergoing a procedure involving removal of a polyp under direct visualisation.

26. A 35-year-old woman presents with a right adnexal mass and free fluid in the pouch of Douglas. Her serum β-hCG is 3500 IU. She has opted for surgical management.

Answers: MCQs

1. A False

    B False

    C False

    D True

    E True

    The risk of bowel injury is about 4/10,000. The risk of damage to major blood vessels is reported as 2/10,000. The risk of major blood vessel injury has not been reported to be reduced by using Hasson technique. It is believed the direct trocar insertion where non-cutting trocars are used under direct laparoscopic vision, do not increase risk of complications. Hasson technique is recommended for both morbidly obese patients and very thin patients.

Answers: SBAs

2. D The overall risk of serious complications is low, approximately 2 in 1000 women

15% of bowel injuries are not diagnosed at the time of laparoscopy. Wound gaping occurs frequently and does not lead to intraperitoneal sepsis. The open technique can be associated with bowel injury. Two trials have compared the open and closed technique, and a meta-analysis does not indicate that one is safer than the other.

The overall risk of serious complications is low (uncommon) quoted as 2:1000. Thin woman carries a higher risk of blood vessel injury during laparoscopy.

3. C 7 in 1000

A return to theatre following a hysterectomy is a serious complication but it is uncommon. A patient may return to theatre because of bleeding or wound dehiscence, which occurs in 7 in every 1000 cases.

4. C Abdominal hysterectomy

Open surgery is associated with a higher risk of infection as compared to laparoscopic or vaginal route.

5. D Vaginal hysterectomy

With abdominal surgery, you are more likely to achieve complete haemostasis as compared to vaginal surgery.

6. C 3–8 in 100000

Death following a diagnostic laparoscopy is extremely rare: approximately 3–8 women in every 100,000 undergoing a laparoscopy die as result of complications.

7. B Inferior epigastric

During the insertion of secondary ports, it is essential that the inferior epigastric vessels are visualised laparoscopically to ensure trocar tip is away from the vessel. The vessels (artery and vein) can be seen just lateral to the lateral umbilical ligaments in most patients.

8. A IAP 20–25 mmHg before the insertion of the primary trocar

Achieving a pressure of 20–25 mmHg before inserting the trocar is necessary because this results in increased splinting and allows the trocar to be more easily inserted through the layers of the abdominal wall. The increased size of the gas bubble and this splinting effect has been shown to be associated with a lower risk of major vessel injury.

9. D Previous caesarean section

These techniques will allow easier access in obese women, reduce risk of vascular injury in very thin women and reduce risk of bowel injury in women with vertical abdominal incision and with multiple laparoscopies.

10. B Thin nulliparous women

The aorta may lie less than 25 mm below the skin in very thin women and use of excess force during entry in women with well-developed abdominal musculature will potentially increase the risk of major vessel injury.

11. B Normal saline has better image quality than CO_2

The significantly increased risk of an unsatisfactory view on hysteroscopy with the use of carbon dioxide is mainly attributed to bubbles and bleeding. Normal saline produces lavage of the cavity and so washes away any blood or mucus which otherwise might obscure the view.

12. B 7 days

Start mechanical venous thromboembolism (VTE) prophylaxis at admission. Add pharmacological VTE prophylaxis for patients who have a low risk of major bleeding, taking into account individual patient factors and clinical judgment. Continue pharmacological VTE prophylaxis until the patient no longer has significantly reduced mobility (generally 5–7 days).

13. B Laparoscopy + salpingectomy

The above scenario likely to suggest ruptured ectopic pregnancy, although no mass identified on scan, the patient condition warrants intervention. Laparoscopy or laparotomy can be suitable options however laparoscopy is favoured over laparotomy if skills are present and patient is suitable.

Answers: EMQs

14. I Thromboembolism

This patient has an elevated body mass index and has had extensive surgery in the pelvis. Prolonged pelvic surgery is a risk factor for venous thromboembolism and this patient should be investigated for a pulmonary embolism.

15. C Bradycardia

Reflex bradycardia after establishment of pneumoperitoneum due to vagal stimulation is a known complication of laparoscopic surgery. This may be more likely in young patients with a low BMI.

16. B Bowel injury

The most common visceral injury at laparoscopic entry is a bowel injury. Her previous surgery and working diagnosis put her at increased risk. The description fits with a small bowel injury.

17. K Uterine perforation

This is a case of uterine perforation that is likely to have occurred during the hysteroscopy but was not recognised.

18. D Inferior epigastric vessel injury

Injury of the inferior epigastric artery is described.

19. C Intramuscular methotrexate

The diagnosis is an ectopic pregnancy and the patient's β-HCG is below 3000 mIU/mL with minimal fluid. In addition, the patient is not keen on surgical treatment. Therefore, intramuscular methotrexate is indicated.

20. E Conservative management

This patient needs to be reassured at this point. Because she is clinically stable and the scan is inconclusive at this stage, she can be managed conservatively. She needs a follow-up with serial β-hCG and a repeat scan in 1 week to identify the location of pregnancy. However, warning signs and symptoms should be explained to her and she should be advised to seek urgent help if needed.

21. G Ultrasound

Although full blood count and urea and electrolytes will be part of her work-up, the question concerns the investigation for a suspected complication. In this scenario, the suspected complication is a haematoma. Ultrasound can help to identify a subcutaneous or intraperitoneal collection as well as can also assist in image-guided aspiration or percutaneous drainage in selected cases. A decision regarding any further management depends on the diagnosis.

22. A CT Urogram

Even though the right ureteric dissection was performed, thermal injury to the ureters is known. There should be high index of suspicion for ureteric injury in this woman given the operative findings and the postoperative complaints.

23. H Bowel injury

Bowel injury incidence is reported to be 0–0.5%. About half of these injuries occur at the time of entry, and the rest during the procedure. Most of the intraoperative injuries are thermal and not diagnosed at the time of surgery. A delayed diagnosis can be life-threatening. Bowel injury is reported to be the most common cause of laparoscopic-related mortality. Use of monopolar thermal energy has an inherent risk of wide thermal spread. This can lead to bowel injury in the surrounding area leading to gradual bowel necrosis, perforation and peritonitis. Bipolar devices and ultrasonic devices are safer as they cause less spread of energy.

24. K Uterine perforation

Perforation of the cervix or uterus can occur with any intrauterine surgery but is more likely during therapeutic rather than diagnostic procedures. Risk factors for perforation include nulliparity, scarring from previous cervical surgery, distortion of uterine anatomy, e.g. extreme retroversion or fibroids and postmenopausal endometrial atrophy. Uterine perforation typically occurs at the fundus which can lead to visceral damage. It can also occur laterally, damaging blood vessels. Signs of this complication include excessive bleeding, sudden loss of visual field or hypotension. The procedure should be immediately stopped and laparoscopy should be performed to visualise uterus, adnexa and bowel to exclude any injury. If the patient is not haemodynamically stable, laparotomy should be performed.

25. I Risk of death (3–8 in 100,000)

3–8 women in every 100,000 undergoing diagnostic hysteroscopy die as a result of complications, and although very rare, this should be discussed during the consent-taking process. Uterine perforation and bleeding are also correct choices, but the most significant complication is death.

26. H Risk of serious complications of 2 in 1000

Failure to gain entry is another correct choice to be included in the consent process, but H is the most specific information that must be included in the consent process.

Chapter 19

Urogynaecology including prolapse

Questions: MCQs

Answer each stem 'True' or 'False'.

1. **The risk of developing pelvic floor prolapse is associated with:**
   - **A**   Obesity
   - **B**   Obstructed defecation
   - **C**   Forceps delivery
   - **D**   Previous hysterectomy
   - **E**   High impact activities

Questions: SBAs

For each question, select the single best answer from the five options listed.

2. A 40-year-old woman with two children reports symptoms of stress urinary incontinence but would like to avoid surgery as she has not completed her family yet.

   Which of the following medication would you prescribe to improve her symptoms?

   A Sertraline
   B Duloxetine
   C Solifenacin
   D Oxybutinin
   E Mirabegron

3. A 70-year-old patient with overactive bladder symptoms undergoes an urodynamic test. She has a first sensation of filling at 70 mL with a concomitant detrusor pressure of 2 cmH$_2$O. The bladder is filled to 300 mL when she reports lower abdominal pain, urgency to pass urine and the filling is stopped. At the end of the cystometry the detrusor pressure of 20 cmH$_2$O and no detrusor overactivity is detected.

   Which of the following descriptions in relation to the above test can be associated lower urinary tract dysfunction and neurological conditions?

   A Relationship between bladder volume and bladder pressure ($\Delta v/\Delta p$)
   B Relationship between bladder pressure and bladder volume ($\Delta p/\Delta v$)
   C Relationship between maximum cystometric capacity and first sensation of filling (MCC/FSF)
   D Relationship between first sensation of filling and maximum cystometric capacity (FSF/MCC)
   E Feeling that leads the patient to pass urine at the next convenient moment

4. A 75-year-old woman complains of frequency, nocturia and urgency, with no episodes of urinary incontinence. The 3-day bladder diary shows she passes urine 5–6 times during the day and once during the night. Urodynamic assessment shows a bladder capacity of 200 mL with no evidence of detrusor overactivity.

   Which of the following statements is correct?

   A The woman can be diagnosed with an overactive bladder despite urodynamic assessment did not show detrusor over-activity
   B The woman does not suffer from nocturia as she voids only once during the night-time
   C A bladder capacity of 200 mL can be considered normal in a postmenopausal patient
   D A bladder capacity of 200 mL is normal regardless the patient age
   E Systemic hormone replacement therapy (HRT) would be more effective than vaginal HRT in this clinical scenario

5. A woman complains of urinary incontinence only when she coughs. Urodynamic assessment shows an increase in the detrusor pressure immediately after coughs with concomitant urinary leakage.

Which is her urodynamic diagnosis?

A Urodynamic stress urinary incontinence
B Overactive bladder
C Cough-provoked detrusor overactivity with associated incontinence
D Mixed urinary incontinence
E Systolic detrusor overactivity

6. A 27-year-old woman has a history of voiding difficulties. At uroflowometry she voids 120 mL of urine with a peak-flow rate of 16 mL/sec, a bell-shaped curve and a post-void residual of 20 mL.

Which of the following is correct?

A The uroflowometry is normal
B The patient peak-flow rate is low and therefore the patient needs further investigations
C The uroflowometry should be repeated as the voided volume should be > 150 mL
D The voiding function is abnormal as the post-void residual is > 15 mL
E The patient should be taught clean intermittent self-catheterisation

7. A reduced bladder compliance can be caused by which of the following:

A Use of antimuscarinics
B Vescico-ureteric reflux
C Bladder diverticula
D Large uterine fibroids
E Urethral diverticulum

8. A patient has a long-standing history of stress-predominant urinary incontinence and frequency. The clinician is thinking of inserting a retropubic tape to treat her stress urinary incontinence, but he would like to exclude any underlying detrusor overactivity (DO).

Which is the most sensitive test to diagnose DO?

A Standard urodynamics off-antimuscarinics
B Standard urodynamics on-antimuscarinics
C Ambulatory urodynamics off-antimuscarinics
D Ambulatory urodynamics on-antimuscarinics
E Frequency-volume chart

9. Which of the following cannot be assessed during filling cystometry?

A Detrusor activity
B Bladder sensation
C Bladder capacity

    D   Bladder compliance
    E   Urethral pressure profile

10. A 40-year-old woman presents with dyspareunia, dysuria and post-void dribbling. She is known to suffer from recurrent urinary tract infections and 2 years previously she had a retropubic tension-free vaginal tape. Videourodynamics is performed.

    Which of the following findings could explain her symptoms?

    A   Vesico-ureteric reflux
    B   Mesh-erosion
    C   Urethral diverticulum
    D   Detrusor overactivity
    E   Vesico-vaginal fistula

11. A 30-year-old nulliparous woman presents with new onset symptoms of overactive bladder. She is known to suffer from diabetes mellitus type 1 since childhood. Urodynamics show a bladder capacity of 300 mL and repetitive detrusor contractions, a maximum detrusor pressure of 120 cmH$_2$O with no associated incontinence.

    Which of the following diagnosis could explain her symptoms?

    A   Urinary tract infection
    B   Bladder calculi
    C   Multiple sclerosis
    D   Vesical endometriosis
    E   Detrusor sphincter dyssynergia

12. A 65-year-old patient presents with new onset symptoms of vaginal swelling, constipation and occasional urinary leakage on exertion. She underwent a colposuspension for stress urinary incontinence few years ago.

    Which of the following can be attributed to her previous continence surgery?

    A   Stress urinary incontinence
    B   Mesh erosion
    C   Nocturia
    D   Cystocoele
    E   Rectocele

13. Which of the following is not a risk factor for genital prolapse?

    A   Hypermobility syndrome
    B   Obesity
    C   Multiple sclerosis
    D   Constipation
    E   Chronic obstructive pulmonary disease

14. Pelvic organ prolapse involves multiple anatomical and functional systems and is commonly associated with gastrointestinal symptoms.

    What is highly unlikely to be caused by prolapse?

    A   Urgency of defecation
    B   Obstructed defecation
    C   Splinting of the perineum
    D   Diarrhoea
    E   Feeling of incomplete emptying

15. Surgery for pelvic organ prolapse can rely on ligament support.

    Which of the following is involved in the 'paravaginal repair'?

    A   Sacrospinous ligament
    B   Uterosacral ligament
    C   Presacral ligament
    D   Arcus tendineus fasciae pelvis
    E   Round ligament

16. McCall's culdoplasty is performed at the time of a vaginal hysterectomy to treat or prevent:

    A   A low cystocele
    B   A high cystocele
    C   A low rectocele
    D   A high rectocele
    E   Stress urinary incontinence

17. When pelvic floor muscle training of a symptomatic pelvic organ prolapse (POP) can be considered?

    A   During pregnancy
    B   Recurrence after POP surgery
    C   Prior to POP surgery
    D   Body mass index greater than 40
    E   All of the above

18. What is the lifetime risk of undergoing a single operation for prolapse or incontinence?

    A   5%
    B   8%
    C   11%
    D   15%
    E   20%

19. Which operation for upper vaginal prolapse (uterine or vault) is associated with a lower rate of recurrence?

    A   Vaginal sacrospinous colpopexy
    B   Sacral colpopexy
    C   High vaginal uterosacral suspension
    D   Transvaginal polypropylene mesh
    E   They all have similar outcomes

20. There is a clear link between vaginal delivery and symptoms and signs of pelvic organ prolapse in urogynaecological patients.

How much is the risk increased when women who had a forceps delivery are compared with women who had a caesarean section?

    A   OR 1.4
    B   OR 3.2
    C   OR 5.1
    D   OR 7.5
    E   OR 8.3

21. The pelvic organ prolapse - quantification (POP-Q) system is an objective site-specific system for describing, quantifying and staging pelvic support in women.

What is used as a fixed point of reference?

    A   Cervix/vaginal vault
    B   Hymen
    C   Ischial spines
    D   Symphisis pubis
    E   There is no reference point

Questions: EMQs

Questions 22 – 23

Option list for Questions 22 – 23:

A Endometriosis
B Pelvic inflammatory disease
C Ovarian cyst
D Irritable bowel syndrome
E Adhesions
F Ureteric stones
G Interstitial cystitis

H Appendicitis
I Constipation
J Psychological
K Musculoskeletal
L Adenomyosis
M Nerve entrapment

For each case described below, choose the single most likely diagnosis from the above list of options. Each option may be used once, more than once, or not at all.

22. A 28-year-old mother of two is referred to you by her general practitioner with a complaint of lower backache. She has had this pain for the last 8 months, after the first birthday of her last child. The pain is present all the time but she feels it increases more around her periods. She has used combined oral contraceptives for years but now her husband has had a vasectomy. She has no significant past medical or surgical history. On further inquiry she complains of getting constipated around her periods which is manageable with laxatives. She also complains of deep dyspareunia on some occasions, especially on the days when her backache is worsened. She has received physiotherapy for her backache without much benefit.

23. A 45-year-old woman presents with a long-standing history of lower abdominal and pelvic pain. On exploring her history, you do not find any relevant information apart from the fact that she has been known to have a moderate uterine prolapse.

Answers: MCQs

1. A True

   B True

   C False

   D True

   E True

   The risk of pelvic floor prolapse (POP) is increased by a multitude of anatomical, physiological, genetic, lifestyle and reproductive factors. Causative factors of POP are categorised as genetic (e.g. tissue defect), nutritional (e.g. obesity), obstetric (e.g. multiple births with large babies), but a forceps delivery itself is not a risk factor. Intervening factors are high impact activities, chronic constipation with straining, chronic cough, vaginal atrophy. A previous hysterectomy is another risk factor.

Answers: SBAs

2. B Duloxetine

It is a selective serotonin and norepinephrine reuptake inhibitor. Its inhibition of presynaptic neuronal reuptake of serotonin and norepinephrine in the central nervous system results in elevated levels of serotonin and norepinephrine in the synaptic cleft. This leads to an increase in the nerve stimulation of the striated urethral sphincter muscle.

3. A Relationship between bladder volume and bladder pressure ($\Delta v/\Delta p$)

It describes the ability of the bladder to stretch in response to an increase in volume of urine. The gradual increase of detrusor pressure can be associated with spinal cord injury, and the terminal increase had an association with a history of treatment to the pelvic cavity.

4. A The woman can be diagnosed with an overactive bladder despite urodynamic assessment did not show detrusor overactivity

The woman can be diagnosed with an overactive bladder (OAB) despite urodynamics did not show detrusor overactivity. OAB is a symptom syndrome defined as 'urgency, with or without urge incontinence, usually with frequency and nocturia'. The presence of detrusor over-activity is not included in the definition of OAB.

5. C Cough-provoked detrusor overactivity with associated incontinence

The presence of detrusor over-activity immediately after a cough is defined as 'cough-provoked detrusor over-activity'. The urinary leakage concomitant with the increase in the detrusor pressure, even after a cough, cannot be defined as stress incontinence.

6. C The uroflowometry should be repeated as the voided volume should be > 150 mL

A voided volume > 150 mL is necessary to ensure accurate, reproducible curves.

7. D Large uterine fibroids

A large bulky fibroid uterus can compress the bladder causing high pressures with small volumes of urine (compliance $= \Delta v/\Delta p$).

8. C Ambulatory urodynamics off-antimuscarinics

Ambulatory urodynamics (UDS) is a functional test of the lower urinary tract where the bladder is naturally filled. This test lasts therefore longer than standard UDS, increasing the chance of detecting detrusor overactivity (DO). Moreover, to increase the detection rate of DO, the patient should be advised to stop antimuscarinics 7 days before the test.

9. E Urethral pressure profile

Urethral pressure profilometry is the exam to assess the intraurethral pressure. Detrusor activity, bladder sensation, bladder capacity and bladder compliance can be evaluated during filling cystometry.

10. C Urethral diverticulum

Urethral diverticula have been historically described with the classic triad of three Ds (e.g. dyspareunia, dysuria and post-void dribbling). Videourodynamics is a sensitive test for urethral diverticula.

11. C Multiple sclerosis

The urodynamic picture with a reduced capacity, repetitive detrusor contractions and high detrusor pressure is suggestive of an underlying neurological condition.

12. E Rectocele

Patient who undergo colposuspension are at increased risk of developing prolapse of the posterior vaginal wall as colposuspension modifies the axis of the vagina raising the pressure on the posterior compartment.

13. C Multiple sclerosis

Obesity, constipation and chronic obstructive pulmonary disease chronically increase the intra-abdominal pressure. Hypermobility syndrome is a connective tissue disorder, which has been associated with severe prolapse symptoms.

14. D Diarrhoea

All other symptoms can be secondary to a rectocele. A prolapse of the posterior compartment can cause difficulties in emptying the bowels, constipation but no diarrhoea.

15. D Arcus tendineus fasciae pelvis

The paravaginal repair aims to reattach the paravaginal connective tissue to arcus tendineus fascia pelvis, thus correcting lateral defects.

16. D A high rectocele

McCall's culdoplasty involves attaching the uterosacral cardinal ligament complex to the peritoneal surface. This helps in closing off the cul-de-sac and supporting the posterior vaginal apex and the vaginal vault.

17. E All of the above

Pelvic floor muscle training represents a conservative management for prolapse and should be always considered and advised during counselling.

18. C 11%

Olson et al. (1997) reported an 11.1% lifetime risk of undergoing a single operation for pelvic organ prolapse and urinary incontinence.

19. B Sacral colpopexy

A 2013 meta-analysis showed that sacral colpopexy has superior outcomes to a variety of vaginal procedures including sacrospinous colpopexy, uterosacral colpopexy and transvaginal mesh.

20. B OR 3.2

A 2015 meta-analysis showed that highest prevalence of prolapse were found in women delivered at least once by forceps. Compared with women in the caesarean section group, the adjusted odds ratios for reporting symptoms of prolapse were 2.4 (95% CI 1.30–4.59) and 3.2 (95% CI 1.65–6.12) in the normal vaginal delivery/vacuum extraction group and forceps group, respectively.

21. B Hymen

The hymen acts as the fixed point of reference throughout the pelvic organ prolapse - quantification (POP-Q) system. In the POP-Q system each point is measured in centimetres above or proximal to the hymen (negative number) or centimetres below or distal to the hymen (positive number) with the plane of the hymen being defined as zero.

Answers: EMQs

22. A Endometriosis

The history goes in favour of endometriosis, most likely to be deep infiltrated type. The symptoms pointing towards this diagnosis are pain worsening around periods, deep dyspareunia and constipation around periods (likely due to pain). The symptoms might have been masked in the past due to combined oral contraceptive use.

23. K Musculoskeletal

Pelvic organ prolapse may be a source of chronic pelvic pain. In a consecutive series of 26 women who had a negative laparoscopy for pelvic pain, and who subsequently underwent an MRI, 20 were found to have injury to the levator ani.

Chapter 20

Gynaecologic oncology

Questions: MCQs

Answer each stem 'True' or 'False'.

1. **Regarding breast cancer:**
   - A   Breast cancer is the most common cancer in women
   - B   The lifetime risk of breast cancer is 1:15
   - C   15% of breast cancer diagnosed before age of 45 years
   - D   The 5-year survival is around 60%
   - E   Survival is less in younger women

2. **Regarding breast cancer in younger women:**
   - A   It has an inferior prognosis
   - B   It is associated with low grade tumour
   - C   It carries low risk of metastasis
   - D   It has a high E2 receptor negative tumour
   - E   7% of all breast cancer cases happen in women under 40 years

3. **Regarding diagnosis of breast cancer during pregnancy:**
   - A   Cytology is not indicated as it is not conclusive due to proliferative changes during pregnancy
   - B   Tumour markers (CA-125/CA15-3/CEA) are very helpful
   - C   Pelvic CT scan and isotope bone scan are recommended to exclude metastasis
   - D   Diagnosis can be delayed
   - E   Core or excisional biopsy can be used to make a diagnosis

4. **Regarding management of breast cancer during pregnancy:**
   - A   Surgical treatment undertaken in all trimester
   - B   Sentinel node assessment is not safe
   - C   Radiotherapy is contraindicated until delivery
   - D   Chemotherapy is contraindicated until delivery
   - E   Pregnancy worsens the prognosis of women diagnosed of breast cancer

5. **Regarding breast cancer postnatally:**
   - A   Breastfeeding should be avoided if woman take trastuzumab
   - B   Tamoxifen is safe during breast-feeding
   - C   Hormonal contraception is contraindicated
   - D   A levonorgestrel-intrauterine system is safe
   - E   Long-term survival after breast cancer is not adversely affected by pregnancy

6. **Regarding gestational trophoblastic disease:**
    A   The most common form of gestational trophoblastic disease is a partial mole
    B   There are 3 types of hydatidiform moles
    C   The risk of an invasive mole is more common in women aged above 40 years
    D   Choriocarcinoma can occur in men
    E   A partial mole often develops when either 1 or 2 sperm cells fertilise an egg cell that contains no nucleus or DNA

7. **Regarding endometrial hyperplasia:**
    A   The risk of cancer progression in simple endometrial hyperplasia is less than 1%
    B   The risk of cancer progression is complex endometrial hyperplasia without atypia is 50%
    C   The risk of cancer progression of atypical endometrial hyperplasia is 70%
    D   Cyclical oral progesterones can be used in the treatment of complex endometrial hyperplasia
    E   Atypical endometrial hyperplasia is usually managed with cyclical oral progesterone or a levonorgestrel-releasing intrauterine system with repeat pipelle biopsy in 3 months

8. **Regarding postmenopausal bleeding:**
    A   The likelihood of finding endometrial cancer in woman referred urgently to clinic for postmenopausal bleed is 10%
    B   A normal endometrial pipelle biopsy excludes endometrial cancer
    C   An endometrial thickness of 3 mm excludes endometrial cancer
    D   A common cause for postmenopausal bleeding is atrophic changes
    E   If a woman had been thoroughly investigated for postmenopausal bleeding 2 years ago and was given the all clear and has a new episode of vaginal bleeding she can be reassured and does not need further investigation

9. **Regarding tumour markers:**
    A   CA-125 is raised in 5% of normal women
    B   CA-125 of 5630 can be due to endometriosis
    C   CA-27.29 can be raised in ovarian cancer
    D   Tumour M2-PK is associated with cervical cancer
    E   Inhibin is associated with Leydig cell tumours

10. **Regarding the pathophysiology of ovarian cancer:**
    A   High-grade serous epithelial ovarian cancer is thought to arise from the peritoneum
    B   Clear cell ovarian tumours are associated with endometriosis
    C   Krukenberg's tumours are often characterised by mucin-secreting signet-ring cells
    D   Mucinous ovarian tumours are associated with endometriosis
    E   *BRCA1* and *BRCA2* are associated with low-grade serous epithelial ovarian cancer

11. **Regarding chemotherapy:**

   A   Carboplatin is frequently associated with hair loss

   B   Cisplatin is frequently associated with hair loss

   C   Platinum-based chemotherapeutic agents target β-tubulin *DNA*

   D   Platinum-based chemotherapeutic agents work by affecting tubulin aggregation

   E   Paclitaxel causes ototoxicity *Neurotoxic*

12. **Regarding radiotherapy in cervical cancer:**

   A   Radiotherapy is a frequent treatment for cervical cancer with stage IA cervical cancer

   B   Paclitaxel is often given with radiotherapy in the treatment of cervical cancer

   C   Brachytherapy is usually given be before external beam radiotherapy in the treatment of cervical cancer

   D   Radiotherapy to the pelvis can cause fibrosis and narrowing of the vagina and dyspareunia

   E   After high dose brachytherapy up to 35% of women will report bladder or bowel side effects

13. **Regarding human papillomavirus (HPV):**

   A   HPV 11 is a high-risk strain causing CIN 3

   B   HPV 18 causes genital warts

   C   HPV 42 is a high-risk strain causing CIN 3

   D   The quadrivalent HPV vaccine protects against HPV strains 6, 12, 16 and 18 *16/18*

   E   The bivalent HPV vaccine protects against HPV strains 6 and 12 *6, 11, 16-18*

14. **Regarding the prognosis of gynaecological cancers in the UK:**

   A   The 5-year survival of stage II endometrial cancer is more than 80% *95*

   B   The 5-year survival of stage IV endometrial cancer is around 15%

   C   The 5-year survival for stage IV cervical cancer is around 15% *75*

   D   The 5-year survival for stage IV ovarian cancer is around 5%

   E   The 5-year survival for stage I ovarian cancer is around 80% *40*

15

Questions: SBAs

For each question, select the single best answer from the five options listed.

15. A 62-year-old woman presents to rapid-access gynaecology clinic with vaginal bleeding. She has a history of breast cancer and had a wide local excision and axillary clearance 8 years ago followed by 5 years of tamoxifen. She has a body mass index (BMI) of 30. Her periods stopped at the age of 50 years and she had 2 years of combined hormone replacement therapy. She is an ex-smoker.

What is the most significant risk factor for endometrial cancer?

    A The patient's history of breast cancer
    B The patient's body mass index
    C The patient's past use of hormone replacement therapy
    D The patient's smoking history
    E The patient's past use of tamoxifen

16. A 54-year-old woman presents with a diagnosis of endometrial cancer. On examination you note multiple skin-tag-like lesions. She has also had recent surgery for a 'growth' on her eye, which she said, was benign but related to the skin lesions. She has a history of breast cancer and underwent a wide local excision and tamoxifen 10 years ago.

Which genetic predisposition is she likely to have?

    A *BRCA1*
    B *BRCA2*
    C Cowden's syndrome
    D Lynch's syndrome
    E Muir–Torre syndrome

17. A 39-year-old woman has a laparoscopic myomectomy for fibroids and subfertility. She is nulliparous and trying for a baby. The histology shows a leiomyosarcoma.

What is the next appropriate step?

    A Total abdominal hysterectomy, bilateral salpingo-oophorectomy and omentectomy
    B Total abdominal hysterectomy with bilateral salpingectomy, omentectomy and ovarian conservation
    C Total laparoscopic hysterectomy with bilateral salpingectomy and ovarian conservation
    D Staging CT chest, abdomen and pelvis and hysterectomy if imaging suggests disease
    E MRI pelvis and staging CT chest and abdomen and hysterectomy if imaging suggests disease

18. A 32-year-old woman seen in colposcopy is diagnosed with squamous cell cervical cancer, width 10 mm, and depth 3 mm. There is no extension to the surrounding structures. She has no children and is keen to preserve her fertility. Her body mass index is 25 and she has no significant co-morbidities.

What is the most appropriate treatment for her?

A Chemoradiotherapy
B Large loop excision of transformation zone
C Radical hysterectomy without lymphadenectomy
D Radical hysterectomy with lymphadenectomy
E Trachelectomy

19. A 68-year-old woman with long-standing lichen sclerosis noticed a new pigmented lesion < 1 cm on her left labium. A punch biopsy confirms differentiated VIN with no evidence of invasion.

What is the most appropriate management for her?

A Clobetasol cream (potent topical steroid)
B Prednisolone (oral steroids)
C Wide local excision
D Wide local excision and sentinel lymph node sampling
E Wide local excision and ipsilateral groin node dissection

20. A 71-year-old woman has developed squamous cell carcinoma of the vulva on a background of Paget's disease. The lesion measures 1 × 5 cm and is located on the right vulva with its innermost margin 2 cm from the midline.

What management would you recommend?

A Radical vulvectomy
B Wide radical excision
C Wide radical excision and sentinel node excision
D Wide radical excision and unilateral groin node surgery
E Wide radical excision and bilateral groin node surgery

Questions: EMQs

Questions 21 – 23

Option list for Questions 21 – 23:

A	Brenner tumour	G	High-grade serous epithelial cancer
B	Choriocarcinoma	H	Leydig cell tumour
C	Clear cell tumour of ovary	I	Mature cystic ovarian teratoma
D	Dysgerminoma	J	Ovarian fibroma
E	Endometriosis	K	Ovarian thecoma
F	Granulosa tumour		

For each of the following cases, select the single most likely diagnosis. Each option may be used once, more than once or not at all.

21. A 45-year-old woman undergoes a total laparoscopic hysterectomy and bilateral salpingo-oophorectomy for endometrial cancer. She has a body mass index of 20 and no relevant medical or family history. At the time of surgery her left ovary has a distinct yellow appearance.

22. An 18-year-old woman with a pelvic mass arising from the right adnexa. Lactate dehydrogenase is markedly elevated.

23. A 48-year-old woman undergoes total laparoscopic hysterectomy and bilateral salpingo-oophorectomy as part of risk-reducing surgery for *BRCA1* mutation. The histology of the ovaries shows occult malignancy.

Questions 24 – 27

Option list for Questions 24 – 27:

A	0	G	255
B	10	H	315
C	40	I	700
D	85	J	2240
E	90	K	2310
F	140	L	4335

For each of the following cases, select the correct risk of malignancy index score. Each option may be used once, more than once or not at all.

24. A 64-year-old postmenopausal woman with bilateral with a left ovarian cyst measuring 4 cm and containing a single septation and a right simple cyst measuring 6 cm. Her CA-125 is 35 kU/L.

25. A 51-year-old woman who is premenopausal has bilateral complex ovarian cysts with multiple septations and solid components. There is also a trace of free fluid and some internal blood flow. Her CA-125 is 85 kU/L.

26. A 42-year-old woman has a 9 cm right fluid-filled ovarian cyst with a thin wall and no solid components. There are no loculations, free fluid or internal blood flow. Her CA-125 is 55 kU/L.

27. A 70-year-old woman has a complex 6 cm ovarian cyst with solid and liquid components and multiple septations. There is a small amount of free fluid. Her CA-125 is 10 kU/L.

Questions 28 – 30

Option list for Questions 28 – 30:

A	Stage IA1	G	Stage IIB1
B	Stage IA2	H	Stage IIIA
C	Stage IB1	I	Stage IIIB
D	Stage IB2	J	Stage IVA
E	Stage IIA1	K	Stage IVB
F	Stage IIA2		

For each of the following clinical findings, select the correct stage from the options listed above. Each option may be used once, more than once or not at all.

28. A 3 cm squamous cell carcinoma of cervix, no extension to uterus, parametria or vagina on imaging or examination under anaesthetic.

29. A large cervical tumour with involvement of the lower third of the vagina, parametria but no bladder or bowel involvement or distant metastasis.

30. A 2 cm cervical tumour but with involvement of upper two thirds of the vagina and parametrial invasion. There is no evidence of extension to pelvic side wall or lower third of vagina or distant organs.

Questions 31 – 34

Option list for Questions 31 – 34:

A	Azathioprine	H	Mycophenolate
B	Canesten cream	I	Prednisolone
C	Cyclosporine	J	Reassurance and counselling to break
D	Clobetasol cream		the itch cycle
E	Imiquimod	K	Wide local excision and groin node
F	Methotrexate		dissection
G	Moisturisers		

For each of the following cases, select the single most appropriate treatment. Each option may be used once, more than once or not at all.

31. A 65-year-old woman has long standing itching of the vulva worse at night. On examination the vulva there is white shiny appearance with loss of labial architecture.

32. A 70-year-old woman presents with a 3 cm squamous cell cancer on her right labia.

33. A 45-year-old woman presents with multicentric VIN. *E*

34. A 50-year-old woman presents with itching and burning of the vulva. On examination there are lacy reticular lesions on the vulva.

Questions 35 – 38

Option list for Questions 35 – 38:

A	Stage IA	H	Stage IIIA1
B	Stage IB	I	Stage IIIA2
C	Stage IC1	J	Stage IIIB
D	Stage IC2	K	Stage IIIC
E	Stage IC3	L	Stage IVA
F	Stage IIA	M	Stage IVB
G	Stage IIB		

For each of the following cases, select the stage. Each option may be used once, more than once or not at all.

35. An 80-year-old woman presents with a large pelvic mass. Imaging reveals liver metastasis and extensive peritoneal deposits with appearances suggestive of omental cake.

36. A 68-year-old woman presents with bilateral ovarian tumours but no evidence of spread elsewhere.

37. A 70-year-old woman presents with high-grade serous ovarian cancer extending into uterus and fallopian tubes. No other pelvic organs are involved and there is no evidence of distant metastasis.

38. A 60-year-old woman presents with high-grade serous ovarian cancer extending into uterus and fallopian tubes. In addition, there are multiple peritoneal deposits > 2 cm in the upper abdomen with evidence of tumour on the surface/capsule of the spleen only.

Questions 39 – 41

Option list for Questions 39 – 41:

A	Oral combined contraceptive pill
B	Surgical treatment late thirties/early forties (bilateral salpingectomy only)
C	Surgical treatment late forties/early fifties (bilateral salpingectomy only)
D	Surgical treatment late fifties/early sixties (bilateral salpingectomy only)
E	Surgical treatment late sixties/early seventies (bilateral salpingectomy only)
F	Surgical treatment late thirties/early forties (bilateral salpingo-oophorectomy)
G	Surgical treatment late forties/early fifties (bilateral salpingo-oophorectomy)

H   Surgical treatment late fifties/
early sixties (bilateral salpingo-
oophorectomy)

I   Surgical treatment late sixties/
early seventies (bilateral salpingo-
oophorectomy)

J   Surgical treatment late thirties/
early forties (total hysterectomy and
bilateral salpingo-oophorectomy)

K   Surgical treatment late forties/early
fifties (total hysterectomy and bilateral
salpingo-oophorectomy)

L   Surgical treatment late fifties/early
sixties (total hysterectomy and
bilateral salpingo-oophorectomy)

M   Surgical treatment late sixties/early
seventies (total hysterectomy and
bilateral salpingo-oophorectomy)

For each of the following cases, select the most appropriate cancer-reducing treatment
and the optimal timing for that treatment. Each option may be used once, more than
once or not at all.

39. A 30-year-old woman is known to have the *BRCA1* mutation. Her sister and mother
died from breast cancer. She is asymptomatic and her family is not complete.

40. A 40-year-old woman is known to have the *BRCA2* mutation. She is asymptomatic
and her family is not complete.

41. A 28-year-old woman has hereditary non-polyposis colorectal cancer (Lynch's
syndrome). She is asymptomatic and family is not complete.

Questions 42 – 44

Option list for Options 42 – 44:

A   Full staging laparotomy in a cancer
centre

B   Laparoscopic aspiration of the cyst

C   Laparoscopic bilateral salpingo-
oophorectomy in a cancer centre

D   Laparoscopic bilateral salpingo-
oophorectomy in a general
gynaecology centre

E   Laparoscopic ovarian cystectomy

F   Laparoscopic unilateral salpingo-
oophorectomy

G   Laparotomy, removal of the ovarian

cyst and frozen section examination
and proceed

H   MRI of pelvis and CA-125 in 1 month

I   MRI of pelvis and CA-125 in 4 months

J   MRI of pelvis and CA-125 in 12
months

K   Ultrasound scan of pelvis and CA-125
in 1 month

L   Ultrasound scan of pelvis and CA-125
in 4 months

M   Ultrasound scan of pelvis and CA-125
in 12 months

For each of the following cases, select the most appropriate treatment. Each option
may be used once, more than once or not at all.

42. A 68-year-old woman has a complex bilateral multiloculated cysts. Her CA-125 is
30 kU/L.

43. A 59-year-old woman has a right enlarged complex ovarian cyst containing 2 thick
walled septa and solid components. There is significant ascites and CT imaging
suggests peritoneal deposits and deposits underneath the diaphragm and near the
sigmoid colon.

44. A 59-year-old woman has a 4.5 cm simple cyst on the left ovary, CA-125 is 10 kU/L.

Questions 45 – 47

Option list for Questions 45 – 47:

A   Additional adhoc cervical smears
B   Annual cervical smears
C   BRCA testing for patient
D   BRCA testing for relative
E   CA-125 blood test
F   No screening is available
G   Pelvic ultrasound
H   Pelvic ultrasound and CA-125 blood test
I   Referral to a genetic counsellor
J   Routine cervical screening

For each of the following cases, select the initial appropriate screening test. Each option may be used once, more than once or not at all.

45. A 30-year-old woman is very anxious because her sister died of cervical cancer aged 33 years.

46. A 45-year-old woman has a sister who has recently been diagnosed with breast cancer, and their mother died of ovarian cancer aged 70 years.

47. A 45-year-old woman who had breast cancer and is *BRCA1* positive wants to know if her ovaries are will be affected.

Answers: MCQs

1. A True

    B False

    C True

    D False

    E True

    The lifetime risk of breast cancer is 1:9. The 5-year survival for breast cancer is around 80%.

2. A True

    B False

    C False

    D True

    E True

    Breast cancer in younger women is more aggressive, associated with high grade tumour, high E2 receptor negative tumour and carries high risk of metastasis.

3. A True

    B False

    C False

    D True

    E True

    Due to proliferative changes during pregnancy, cytology is not indicated. Tumour markers during pregnancy are misleading and not helpful therefore not recommended. Pelvic CT/isotope bone scans used outside pregnancy to exclude metastasis. However, during pregnancy they are not recommended. If bone metastasis is suspected, plain film and MRI should be used instead. There is often a delay in diagnosis in pregnancy due to changes in breast tissue.

4. A True

    B False

    C True

    D False

    E False

    Surgical treatment is undertaken in all trimesters; however reconstruction should be delayed. Sentinel node assessment is safe, but blue dye is not recommended. Radiotherapy is contraindicated until delivery; used only if life-saving or to preserve organ function.

Chemotherapy is contraindicated in 1st trimester, but it is safe after that. There is no evidence for increased rate of miscarriage, fetal growth restriction or organ dysfunction. Pregnancy itself does not worsen the prognosis for women diagnosed in pregnancy compared to non-pregnant controls matched for age and stage (provided standard treatment guidelines are adhered to).

5. A **True**

    B **False**

    C **True**

    D **False**

    E **True**

Breast-feeding should be avoided if woman take trastuzumab or tamoxifen, as these cause neonatal leucopenia. Hormonal contraception is contraindicated (UK cat IV). Regarding levonorgestre-intrauterine system (LNG-IUS), there is no overall increased risk of recurrence but further evidence is needed on its safety. There is increased risk of recurrence in women who developed cancer while using LNG-IUS and continued its use.

6. A **False**

    B **False**

    C **True**

    D **True**

    E **False**

Gestational trophoblastic disease is a group of rare tumours that begin in the trophoblast. There are five main types: hydatidiform mole, invasive mole, choriocarcinoma, placental site trophoblastic tumour and epitheloid trophoblastic tumour. Hydatidiform moles are the most common type and are not malignant. They can be either complete or partial. A complete mole most often develops when either one or two sperm cells fertilise an egg cell that contains no nucleus or DNA. A partial hydatidiform mole develops when two sperm fertilise a normal egg. The treatment of choice for both is an evacuation of retained products of conception. When a hydatidiform mole grows into the myometrium it is called an invasive mole. Complete moles more commonly lead to invasive moles. Choriocarcinoma can either be gestational (often starting off as molar pregnancies) or unrelated to pregnancies, hence can occur in men. Non-gestational choriocarcinomas are more aggressive and less responsive to chemotherapy.

7. A **True**

    B **False**

    C **False**

    D **True**

    E **False**

The risks of cancer progression for simple endometrial hyperplasia, complex endometrial hyperplasia and atypical endometrial hyperplasia are < 1%, 3% and 30% respectively.

A levonorgestrel-releasing intrauterine system or cyclical oral progesterones can be used in the treatment of simple or complex endometrial hyperplasia. For hyperplasia with atypia the management is the same as endometrial cancer as early endometrial cancer is found in up to 50% of cases. An MRI and chest X-ray should be requested and the patient should be reviewed in the gynaeoncology multidisciplinary team with a view to a hysterectomy if there are no fertility considerations.

8. A True

    B False

    C False

    D True

    E False

Approximately 10% of patients presenting with postmenopausal bleeding will have a gynaecological malignancy. Other causes of bleeding include atrophic changes, hyperplasia and polyps. The incidence of endometrial cancer in women with endometrial thickness < 4 mm is 0.6% not zero. Similarly, a pipelle biopsy has a sensitivity of over 90% so a normal result is reassuring but no test excludes malignancy 100%. Subsequently if a patient has new episodes of vaginal bleeding repeat investigations are warranted.

9. A False

    B True

    C True

    D True

    E False

CA-125 is increased in 80% of ovarian cancers but is only sensitive for 50% of stage II cancers. It is raised in 1% of normal women. It is non-specific and raised in breast and colon cancer, fibroids, adenomyosis and endometriosis amongst other things. α-fetoprotein is produced by yolk sac tumours. β-hCG is particularly important for choriocarcinomas. Inhibin is produced by granulosa theca cell tumours. Lactate dehydrogenase may be elevated in some germ cell tumours such as dysgerminoma. CA 27.29 is primarily associated with breast cancer but is also associated prostate, ovarian and colonic cancer. Tumour M2-PK is associated with colorectal cancer, breast cancer, renal cancer, cervical and ovarian cancer

10. A False

    B False

    C True

    D False

E False

A Krukenberg's tumour refers to an ovarian malignancy that has metastasised from a primary site, classically the gastrointestinal tract, although it can arise in other tissues such as the breast. Endometriosis is associated with clear cell ovarian tumours and endometroid ovarian tumours, as is hereditary non-polyposis colorectal cancer. *BRCA1* and *BRCA2* are associated with high-grade serous epithelial ovarian cancer, but not low grade. High-grade serous epithelial ovarian cancer has a precursor lesion on the distal fallopian tube.

11. A False

  B False

  C False

  D False

  E False

Platinum-based chemotherapeutic agents target DNA and cause DNA adduction. They can cause hepatotoxicity, vomiting, renal toxicity, ototoxicity, myelosupression and anaphylaxis.

Paclitaxel acts on β-tubulin and causes tubulin aggregation. It can cause hair loss, neurotoxicity and myelosupression.

12. A False

  B False

  C False

  D True

  E True

Ionising radiation is used in radiotherapy. There are two main forms: external beam radiotherapy (EBRT) and internal radiotherapy (brachytherapy). In cervical cancer (Stage IB2 and above), chemoradiotherapy is used. The chemotherapeutic agent used in cervical cancer with radiotherapy is usually cisplatinum which is given weekly throughout treatment. A course of external radiotherapy is also used which usually lasts 5 weeks. In EBRT high-energy X-rays (or occasionally gamma-rays from a radioisotope like cobalt-60) are directed at the cancer from outside the body. Brachytherapy is then given within 1–2 weeks of completing EBRT. Brachytherapy involves the placement of short-range radioisotopes (usually iridium or cobalt) at the site of the cancerous tumour. These are enclosed in a protective capsule or wire, which allows the ionising radiation to escape to treat and kill surrounding tissue but prevents the charge of radioisotope from moving or dissolving in body fluids.

Frequent side effects post radiotherapy include: nausea, diarrhoea, vaginal and vulval discomfort, vaginal bleeding and bladder irritability. In the long term it can cause early menopause, fibrosis and narrowing of the vagina, vaginal dryness and long-term bladder and bowel symptoms.

13. **A** False

   B False

   C False

   D False

   E False

There are a number of different human papillomavirus (HPV) strains. HPV 6 and 11 manifest as genital warts. HPV 16, 18, 31, 33, 35, 39, 45, 51, 52, 56, 58, 59, 68, 73, 82 are high-risk strains associated with CIN 3. The bivalent vaccine Cervarix protects against HPV 16 and 18. The quadrivalent vaccine Gardisil protects against strains 6, 11, 16 and 18.

14. **A** False

   B True

   C False

   D True

   E False

The prognosis of endometrial cancer will also depend on the type, grade of cancer.

In general, the approximate 5-year survival of endometrial cancer is 95%, 75%, 40% and 15% for stage I, II, III and IV disease respectively. Statistics are taken from Cancer Research UK.

The 5-year survival for cervical cancer is approximately 96%, 54%, 38% and 5% for stage I, II, III and IV disease respectively. Statistics taken from Anglia Cancer Network.

The 5-year survival for ovarian cancer is approximately 90%, 43%, 19% and 4% for stage I, II, III and IV disease respectively. Statistics taken from Anglia Cancer Network.

The 5-year survival for vulval cancer internationally [data taken from the International Federation of Gynaecological Oncologists (FIGO)] is 80%, 60%, 40% and 15% for stage I, II, III and IV disease respectively.

Answers: SBAs

15. D Her smoking history

Whilst hormone replacement therapy, smoking and raised body mass index are all associated with endometrial cancer, in this scenario the strongest risk factor for endometrial cancer is tamoxifen use. Tamoxifen is a selective oestrogen receptor modulator and if taking for more than 2 years increases risk of endometrial cancer substantially.

16. C Cowden syndrome

BRCA1 and *BRCA2* mutations are associated with a life-time risk of ovarian cancer of 50% and 30% respectively. Hereditary non-polyposis colorectal cancer, so known as Lynch's syndrome, is due to a fault in mismatch repair genes and is associated with colon cancer, endometrial, ovarian cancer, stomach cancer, pancreatico-biliary, urinary tract and glioblastoma. Cowden syndrome is associated with multiple hamartomas (as described above) and both breast and endometrial cancer.

17. A abdominal hysterectomy, bilateral salpingo-oophorectomy and omentectomy

Leiomyosarcomas account for 3–7% of uterine malignancies. If an unexpected diagnosis of a leiomyosarcoma is made after a myomectomy, full surgical staging is recommended. Ovarian metastases do occur and some sarcomas express oestrogen receptors. Adjuvant therapy includes chemotherapy and radiotherapy. However, pelvic radiotherapy has demonstrated a reduction in local recurrence but not overall survival.

18. D Radical hysterectomy with lymphadenectomy

She has stage IB disease as the lateral spread of tumour is more than 7 mm. Therefore, treatment of choice would be radical hysterectomy and lymphadenectomy. Fertility preserving surgery (trachelectomy) is an option for earlier disease, stage IA2 disease. Chemoradiotherapy could also be used, but given the size of the tumour, lack of co-morbidities and age surgery would be preferable.

19. C Wide local excision

Lichen sclerosus is treated with topical potent steroids. The risk of lichen sclerosus resulting in squamous cell carcinoma is approximately 5%. Vulval intraepithelial neoplasia (VIN) is divided into usual type VIN (often associated HPV) and differentiated VIN that is often associated vulval dermatological conditions. Treatment is always recommended for VIN and incudes: wide local excision, laser ablation or medical therapy (e.g. imiquimod). Removal of groin nodes is essential part of treatment for vulval cancer but not VIN.

20. E Wide radical excision and bilateral groin node surgery

This lesion is more than 2 cm and therefore groin node surgery is important (if depth of invasion is greater than 1 mm, i.e. FIGO stage IB or worse same applies). As the tumour is > 4 cm in maximum diameter it is not suitable for sentinel lymph node excision. Regarding whether unilateral or bilateral groin node excision is required this will depend on the location of the tumour. If it is lateral a unilateral groin node excision is acceptable. A lateral tumour is one in which the wide excision, at least 1 cm beyond the visible tumour edge, would not impinge upon a midline structure (clitoris, urethra, vagina, perineal body, anus). However, one must keep in mind that for a wide local excision you need at least a minimum margin of 15 mm of disease-free tissue on all margins. Therefore, in this particular case by the time a 15-mm margin is excised the margin of excision will be 5 mm from midline making it a midline tumour and warranting bilateral lymph node dissection.

Answers: EMQs

21. F Granulosa cell tumour

These secrete oestrogen and have a yellowish appearance. They are frequently unilateral. As they produce oestrogen women can present with irregular bleeding or may even have concomitant endometrial cancer (as in this case).

22. D Dysgerminoma

These tumours are often unilateral and present in young women. Lactate dehydrogenase is a common tumour marker.

23. G High-grade serous epithelial ovarian cancer

This is the most common ovarian cancer overall and is associated with *BRCA* mutations.

24. H 315

See **Table 20.1.**

Table 20.1 Calculation of the risk of malignancy index (RMI)
$$RMI = M \times U \times C$$
where:
M is menopausal status: premenopausal =1, postmenopausal = 3
C is the CA-125 level
U is the number of suspicious ultrasound features (bilateral, solid areas, multilocular, ascites, evidence of metastasis): if there are none then U = 0; if there is one then U = 1; and if there are two or more suspicious features, U = 3.
Example: simple cysts with no suspicious features has U = 0, therefore RMI = 0
FIGO, the International Federation of Gynaecological Oncologists.

25. G 255

See **Table 20.1.**

26. A 0

See **Table 20.1.**

27. E 90

See **Table 20.1**.

28. C Stage IB1

See **Table 20.2**.

Stage	Extent of disease	5–year survival
\multicolumn{3}{l}{**Table 20.2 FIGO tables of classifications**}
0	Carcinoma in situ	~100%
I	Limited to cervix	
Ia1	Microscopic disease: stromal invasion <3 mm, lateral spread <7 mm	>95%
Ia2	Microscopic disease: stromal invasion <3 mm and >5 mm, lateral spread <7 mm	
Ib1	Macroscopic lesion <4 cm in greatest dimension	90%
Ib2	Macroscopic lesion >4 cm in greatest dimension	80–86%
II	Extension to uterus/parametria/vagina	~75–78%
IIa1	Involvement of upper two thirds of vagina without parametrial invasion, <4 cm greatest diameter	
IIb1	Involvement of upper two thirds of vagina with parametrial invasion	
III	Extension to pelvic side wall and/or lower third of vagina	~47–50%
IIIa	Involvement of lower third of vagina	
IIIb	Extension to palvic side wall and/or hydronephrosis	
IV	Extension to adjacent organs or beyond true pelvis	~20–30%
IVa	Extension to adjacent organs, e.g. bladder, bowel	
IVb	Distant metastases	

29. H Stage IIIA

See **Table 20.2**.

30. G Stage IIB1

See **Table 20.2**.

31. D Clobetasol cream (topical steroid)

The appearances described are characteristic of lichen sclerosus. The treatment of choice is potent steroid cream.

32. K Wide local excision and groin node dissection

This lesion is more than 2 cm, therefore groin node surgery is important (if depth of invasion is >1 mm, i.e. FIGO stage IB or worse, the same applies). As the tumour is > 4 cm in maximum diameter, it is not suitable for sentinel lymph node excision.

Regarding whether unilateral or bilateral groin node excision is required depends on the location of the tumour: if it is lateral a unilateral groin node excision is acceptable. A lateral tumour is one in which the wide excision, at least 1 cm beyond the visible tumour edge, would not impinge upon a midline structure (clitoris, urethra, vagina, perineal body, anus). However, one must keep in mind that for a wide local excision you need at least a minimum margin of 15 mm of disease-free tissue on all margins. Therefore, in this particular case by the time a 15-mm margin is excised the margin of excision will be 5 mm from the midline, making it a midline tumour and warranting bilateral lymph node dissection.

33. E Imiquimod

The treatment of VIN can be wide local excision (no need for lymph nodes), ablation, or medical treatment with imiquimod.

34. I Prednisolone (oral steroid)

The appearance of the vulva is suggestive of lichen planus. A biopsy would be appropriate. Mucosal surfaces can be affected including the mouth. Treatment is with oral steroids.

35. M Stage IVB

See **Table 20.1**.

36. B Stage IB

See **Table 20.1**.

37. F Stage IIA

See **Table 20.1**.

38. K Stage IIIC

See **Table 20.1**.

39. F Surgical treatment late thirties/early forties (bilateral salpingo-oophorectomy)

The current treatment of choice is to remove ovaries and tubes. The mean age for developing ovarian cancer with a *BRCA1* mutation is 51 years old.

40. G Surgical treatment late forties/early fifties (bilateral salpingo-oophorectomy)

The current treatment of choice is to remove the ovaries and tubes. The mean age for developing ovarian cancer with a *BRCA2* mutation is 58 years.

41. J Surgical treatment late thirties/early forties (total hysterectomy and bilateral salpingo-oophorectomy)

In woman with hereditary non-polyposis colorectal cancer (HNPCC), endometrial cancer presents approximately 15 years younger than the usual age of presentation, i.e. post-menopause. It is important for all women with a genetic predisposition to see a genetic counselor prior to treatment. The combined contraceptive pill reduces the risk of ovarian cancer, however surgery is the definitive treatment of choice for risk reduction. Surgery compromises a bilateral salpingo-oophorectomy once a patient's family is complete. One could consider bilateral salpingectomy and delayed oophorectomy in view of current evidence that the fallopian tube is the source of high-grade serous ovarian cancer if the patient is very young though this is not gold standard. For women with HNPCC, because of the strong risk of endometrial cancer a hysterectomy and bilateral salpingo-oophorectomy is recommended. Studies have suggested that the chance of occult cancer being detected at the time of risk-reducing surgery is approximately 5%.

42. G Laparotomy, removal of the ovarian cyst and frozen section examination and proceed

The RMI score is 270 and therefore falls into the high risk category. However, as the imaging does not suggest advanced cancer, laparotomy and frozen section is appropriate. If the mass is non-cancerous a bilateral salpingo-oophorectomy and a hysterectomy will be performed. If the mass is cancerous full staging will be performed including a total hysterectomy, bilateral salpingo-oophorectomy, omentectomy, lymphadenectomy and resection of any peritoneal deposits.

43. A Full staging laparotomy in a cancer centre

This case is suggestive of advanced ovarian malignancy and warrants full staging laparotomy and cytoreductive surgery in a cancer centre.

44. L Ultrasound scan of pelvis and CA-125 in 4 months

A simple unilateral, unilocular cyst < 5 cm with normal CA-125 can be measured conservatively as the risk of cancer is less than 1%. A repeat ultrasound and CA-125 in 4 months is reasonable management. In premenopausal women with simple cysts < 5 cm these are usually functional and over half of these cyst will resolve in 3 months and need no further imaging.

The risk of malignancy score can be used to triage woman for surgery. A low score is one with an RMI < 25 and the risk of cancer is < 3%, these women can therefore have a laparoscopic bilateral salpingo-oophorectomy in a general gynaecology centre. For women with an RMI > 250 this is deemed high risk with a risk of cancer of approximately 75% and warrant a full staging laparotomy. If the RMI score is between 25–250 this is moderate risk of cancer (approximately 20%) and should be managed in a cancer unit. Laparoscopic bilateral salpingo-oophorectomy is acceptable in selected cases.

45. J Routine cervical screening

There is no additional precaution except encouraging her to attend her routine cervical screen invitations, encourage no smoking and to see her general practitioner if she experiences post coital bleeding.

46. I Referral to a genetic counsellor

In the UK, if a first degree relative has cancer and has been diagnosed with *BRCA1* or *BRCA2*, a patient can be referred to a genetic counsellor for *BRCA* testing.

47. F No screening is available

In view of this woman's genetic predisposition, she is at high risk of ovarian cancer. No screening modality has proven so far to be effective for ovarian cancer. She should be referred to a gynaecologic oncologist for discussion for surgical risk reducing surgery.

Chapter 21

Life course approach in gynaecology

Questions: SBAs

For each question, select the single most appropriate answer from the five options listed.

1. A 66-year-old woman presents to the rapid-access gynaecology clinic with a small episode of postmenopausal bleeding. A pelvic ultrasound (transvaginal) scan shows an endometrial thickness of 12 mm but no polyps or fibroids, and her adnexa looks normal. A pelvic examination shows atrophic changes but is otherwise normal. A pipelle biopsy reveals scanty endometrial cells only but no neoplasia, hyperplasia or atypia.

    What is the single most appropriate management step?

    A   Discharge back to the general practitioner with topical hormone replacement therapy (HRT) and instruct her to return if bleeding persists
    B   Discharge back to the general practitioner with oral HRT and instruct her to return if bleeding persists
    C   Hysteroscopy +/– biopsy
    D   Hysterectomy
    E   Repeat ultrasound +/– pipelle biopsy in 3 months

2. A 42-year-old nulliparous woman with a body mass index of 37 presents to the clinic with intermenstrual bleeding and menorrhagia. She is currently trying for a baby. She smokes, has type 2 diabetes and is on metformin. She has a history of migraine. An ultrasound scan showed 2 × 3 cm fundal fibroid, 3 × 3 cm intramural fibroid and a 1 × 2 cm posterior serosal fibroid. Her smears are up-to-date and normal. A pipelle sample shows complex hyperplasia without atypia.

    What is the most appropriate initial treatment option for her?

    A   Combined oral contraceptive and repeat pipelle biopsy in 3 months
    B   Cyclical medroxyprogesterone and repeat pipelle biopsy in 3 months
    C   Hysterectomy with ovarian conservation.
    D   A levonorgestrel-releasing intrauterine system and repeat pipelle biopsy in 3 months
    E   Weight loss and repeat pipelle biopsy in 3 months

3. A patient with postmenopausal bleeding undergoes a transvaginal scan which shows endometrial thickness of 12 mm. The endometrial biopsy is normal.

    What is most appropriate next course of action?

    A   Reassure the patient and discharge her
    B   Repeat biopsy
    C   Hysteroscopy
    D   Hysterectomy
    E   Endometrial ablation

Answers: SBAs

1. C Hysteroscopy +/– biopsy

The main role for investigating postmenopausal bleeding is to diagnose endometrial cancer. The risk of endometrial cancer is < 1% with an endometrial thickness < 4 mm. An ultrasound test is often used as the initial test and most women can be reassured with a normal ultrasound. However, a raised endometrial thickness does raise the prospect of endometrial cancer. Pipelle sampling has a tissue yield failure rate of 7–10% and therefore if the endometrium is markedly thickened a hysteroscopy would be indicated. If the hysteroscopy confirms an atrophic uterine cavity, then topical hormone replacement therapy can be given.

2. B Cyclical medroxyprogesterone and repeat pipelle biopsy in 3 months

Up to 70% of patients may undergo spontaneous regression of complex endometrial hyperplasia without atypia in the absence of ongoing oestrogenic stimulation. However, regression rates of over 90% are seen with both oral progestogens and a levonorgestrel-releasing intrauterine system. Though this patient is trying for a baby, one would recommend weight loss and cyclical progesterones. In view of her body mass index and history of migraines, she would not be suitable for combined oral contraceptive pill. Weight loss would be recommended but it unlikely that she will lose substantial weight in 3 months. A hysterectomy would also be an option if her family was complete. A levonorgestrel-releasing intrauterine system may not be suitable due to distortion of her uterine cavity. After 3 months of treatment repeat sampling is recommended to check for regression.

3. C Hysteroscopy

Hysteroscopy needs to be performed to exclude the possibility of endometrial polyps.

Chapter 22

Sexual health

Questions: MCQs

Answer each stem 'True' or 'False'.

1. The following organisms cause abnormal vaginal discharge:
   A   Gardinella vaginalis
   B   Mycoplasma hominis
   C   Candida glabrata
   D   Group B Streptococcus
   E   Bacterial vaginosis associated bacterium 1

2. Bacterial vaginosis:
   A   Is encountered in all age groups
   B   Is more prevalent in African Americans than Caucasians
   C   Is predominantly caused by an overgrowth of aerobic organisms *anaerobic*
   D   Lactobacilli count remains unchanged
   E   Approximately 50% women are asymptomatic

3. Regarding Trichomoniasis vaginalis:
   A   It is an anaerobic bacterium *protozoa*
   B   It is exclusively sexually transmitted
   C   Urethral infections may be present in up to 90% of episodes
   D   It causes vulval erythema
   E   It causes a fishy smelling discharge

4. Regarding candidiasis:
   A   The majority of women are asymptomatic carriers *20/*
   B   Up to 75% women experience at least one episode during their lifetime
   C   Sexual intercourse increases the risk of infection
   D   Characteristically, it causes satellite skin lesions
   E   Women presenting with dyspareunia should be screened for candidiasis

5. Regarding vaginal discharge:
   A   Bacterial vaginosis is associated with post abortion endometritis
   B   There is increased risk of pre-term birth with bacterial vaginosis
   C   Bacterial vaginosis increase risk of acquiring genital herpes
   D   Vaginal trichomoniasis is associated with pre-term delivery
   E   Routine screening of the male partner is recommended when a woman presents with candidiasis

6.   **Regarding laboratory-based diagnosis of bacterial vaginosis:**
   - A   A curdy white clear, non-smelly discharge
   - B   pH of the vaginal discharge > 6
   - C   Pseudohyphae on gram staining
   - D   Direct observation of the organism on wet microscopy
   - E   A Nugent score of > 4

7.   **Treatment of vaginal discharge**
   - A   Treatment of bacterial vaginosis with vaginal clindamycin cream is more effective than treatment with oral metronidazole
   - B   Treatment of bacterial vaginosis with oral metronidazole for 7 days has a success rate between 60–88%
   - C   Treatment of sexual partners of a woman presenting with *Trichomonas vaginalis* should also be carried out
   - D   Intravaginal and oral treatments of candidiasis are equally effective
   - E   Metronidazole should not be used during first trimester pregnancy because of its teratogenic effects

Questions: SBAs

For each question, select the single best answer from the five options listed.

8. A 25-year-old sexually active woman presents with pelvic pain and vaginal discharge. A urine pregnancy test is negative. On examination, cervical excitation is noted. Vaginal swabs are taken.

    What is the most appropriate next course of action while waiting for the swab results?

    A   Await results and do nothing
    B   Reassure patient and discharge
    C   Start empirical antibiotics
    D   Provide pain relief and reassure the patient that non-steroidal anti-inflammatory drugs should resolve the symptoms
    E   Arrange laparoscopy

9. A 22-year–old woman attends the consultant antenatal clinic at 8 weeks of pregnancy. She has a history of syphilis which was treated 5 years ago. The results of serologic tests for syphilis are as follows:

    Non-treponemal test (rapid plasma reagin assay): non-reactive

    Treponemal test (*Treponema pallidum* particle agglutination assay): reactive

    Which of the following statements is correct?

    A   The baby is at high risk for congenital syphilis
    B   No further action is required
    C   Oral prophylactic erythromycin should be given during pregnancy
    D   The patient needs a lumbar puncture and a venereal disease research laboratory test for her cerebrospinal fluid for neurosyphilis
    E   The patient needs to be checked for syphilis serology IgG

Questions: EMQs

Questions 10 – 13

Option list for Questions 10 – 13:

A   Advise to stop smoking
B   No need for follow up
C   Repeat smear in 1 year
D   Repeat smear in 2 years
E   Repeat smear in 3 years
F   Repeat smear in 5 years
G   Repeat smear in next couple of weeks
H   Refer to colposcopy
I   Refer to genitourinary medicine or sexual health clinic
J   Urgent referral for suspected cancer to colposcopy '2-week wait'

For each of the following cases, select the most appropriate next management step. Each option may be used once, more than once or not at all.

10. A 33-year-old woman was called for routine recall for her smear, however the sample was inadequate. She is a smoker.

11. A 40-year-old woman has a smear which is reported as borderline but is HPV positive.

12. A 48-year-old woman has a smear showing possible glandular disease.

13. A 38-year-old woman has a smear test that shows severe dyskaryosis, suggestive of high-grade cervical intraepithelial neoplasia.

Answers: MCQs

1. A True

    B True

    C True

    D True

    E True

    Bacterial vaginosis is the most common cause of vaginal discharge, caused by *Gardnerella vaginalis*. Recently, bacterial identification using polymerase chain reaction test has identified high prevalence of overgrowth of previously uncultivated bacteria such as bacterial vaginosis associated bacterium (BVAB) 1, 2 and 3 and *Atopobium*. *Mycoplasma hominis* also changes vaginal pH and increase vaginal discharge. *Candida glabrata* is a cause of thrush in about 10% cases. Group B *Streptococcus* infection in the vagina lowers the count of *Lactobacilli* and creates inflammatory conditions.

2. A False

    B True

    C False

    D False

    E True

    Bacterial vaginosis is mainly seen in sexually active women and may also be encountered in menopausal women. It is rather rare in children. It is more prevalent in African Americans and black Africans. It is predominantly caused by anaerobic organisms. There is a change of pH and *Lactobacilli* disappear. Up to 50% of women may be asymptomatic.

3. A False

    B True

    C True

    D True

    E False

    Trichomonas vaginalis is a flagellated protozoon which is a parasite of the genital tract. It is transmitted exclusively by sexual intercourse. During any acute episode, urethral infection is present in 90% of patients but the urinary tract is the sole site of infection in < 5% of cases. A fishy smelling discharge is present in infections with bacterial vaginosis whereas vaginal discharge with trichomoniasis has an offensive smell. Trichomoniasis causes vulval irritation and itching.

4. A False

    B True

    C False

    D True

    E True

Up to 20% women may be asymptomatic and this may rise to up to 40% during pregnancy. It has been estimated that 75% women will experience at least one episode during their life time. Its incidence is not affected by the coital activity rather by other factors such as prolonged treatment with antibiotics, steroids, uncontrolled diabetes mellitus or underlying immunodeficiency. *Candida* infection causes satellite skin lesions, vulval fissuring, vulval erythema and superficial dyspareunia.

5. A True

    B False

    C True

    D False

    E False

There is an association with bacterial vaginosis and post-abortion endometritis. The presence of bacterial vaginosis does increase risk of acquiring sexually transmitted diseases, especially genital herpes and HIV. There is insufficient evidence to show that the treatment of bacterial vaginosis or trichomoniasis influences the pre-term birth rate. Male partners of women presenting with candidiasis do not need to be screened.

6. A False

    B False

    C False

    D False

    E False

The discharge in bacterial vaginosis infection is fishy smelling whereas a curdy discharge is seen in candidiasis. The pH of the vaginal secretions should be > 4.5. Pseudohyphae are diagnostic of candidiasis whereas bacterial vaginosis is diagnosed by seeing clue cells and not the actual bacteria. *Trichomonas vaginalis* can be observed on the wet slide.

7. A False

    B True

    C True

    D True

    E False

Metronidazole and clindamycin have equal efficacy for the treatment of bacterial vaginosis and cure rates reported in various studies varies between 58% and 88% after 1 week's treatment. Partners of women who are being treated for trichomoniasis should also be treated and sexual contact avoided.

Intravaginal and oral routes for candidiasis treatments are equally effective. Metronidazole is neither teratogenic or have a mutagenic effect in infants. It can be used during the first trimester of pregnancy.

Answer: SBAs

8. C Start empirical antibiotics

Empirical treatment is now recommended for suspected pelvic inflammatory disease (PID) due to the low sensitivity and specificity of clinical diagnosis and the associated high morbidity. It is likely that delaying treatment increases the risk of the PID becoming worse, and also the risk of future complications (such as ectopic pregnancy, subfertility or chronic pelvic pain).

9. B No further action is required

The results suggest successful treatment to previous infection. Detection of antibodies to non-treponemal antigens, such as cardiolipin (a lipoidal antigen released by host cells damaged by *Treponema pallidum*) may help to differentiate between active and past syphilis infection. Non-treponemal antibodies are detected by the rapid plasma reagin (RPR) assay, which is typically positive during current infection and negative following treatment or during late/latent forms of syphilis.

For prenatal syphilis screening, the syphilis IgG test (SYPGN/syphilis antibody, IgG, serum) is recommended. Testing for IgM-class antibodies to *Treponema pallidum* should not be performed during routine pregnancy screening unless clinically indicated.

Historically, the serologic testing algorithm for syphilis included an initial non-treponemal screening test, such as the RPR assay or the venereal disease research laboratory (VDRL) tests. Because these tests measure the host's antibody response to non-treponemal antigens, they may lack specificity. Therefore, a positive result by RPR or VDRL requires confirmation by a treponemal-specific test, such as the fluorescent treponemal antibody-absorbed (FTA-ABS) or the *Treponema pallidum* particle agglutination (TP-PA). Although the FTA-ABS and TP-PA are technically simple to perform, they are labour-intensive and require subjective interpretation by testing personnel.

Answers: EMQs

10. G Repeat smear in next couple of weeks

Three consecutive inadequate smears would prompt referral to colposcopy.

11. H Refer to colposcopy

12. J Urgent referral for suspected cancer to colposcopy '2-week wait'

Other indications for urgent referral include an abnormal cervix and evidence of invasive disease.

13. H Refer to colposcopy

If high-grade cervical intraepithelial neoplasia confirmed, in most cases treatment such as large loop excision of transformation zone would be offered.

Section C

Mock papers

Chapter 23

Mock paper 1: obstetrics

Question: MCQs

Answer each stem 'True' or 'False'.

1. Adverse outcomes seen among pregnant teenage mothers are:
   - x A   Higher maternal mortality rates
   - x B   Infant mortality is 100% higher compared with mothers between 25 and 30 years of age
   - C   More likely to suffer from postpartum depression
   - x D   More likely to have higher incidence of large-for-date babies
   - E   Infants are likely to have higher risk of central nervous system congenital anomalies

2. In postpartum pyrexia, increased incidence of maternal sepsis is attributed to:
   - x A   Young age at first pregnancy
   - x B   Hypothyroidism
   - x C   The enhanced virulence of circulating Group D *Streptococcus*
   - D   Non-white Caucasians
   - E   Major postpartum haemorrhage

3. Regarding group A *Streptococcus pyogenes* (GAS):
   - x A   About 20% of all GAS infections manifest as puerperal sepsis   2/.
   - x B   GAS is commonly acquired in hospital
   - C   Patients infected with GAS often present with a sore throat
   - x D   GAS is an uncommon cause of maternal mortality
   - x E   GAS infection usually occurs antenatally

4. The following are classical signs of septicaemic shock:
   - x A   A pulse rate > 200 beats/min
   - x B   A respiratory rate > 30 breaths/min
   - C   A temperature < 35°C
   - x D   A systolic blood pressure 110 mmHg or below
   - x E   A urinary output < 5 mL/kg/hr

5. The following preventive intervention can reduce the risk of sepsis during pregnancy and puerperium:
   - x A   Oral erythromycin for women with preterm labour
   - x B   Women with positive group B *Streptococcus* vaginal swab during pregnancy being treated with antibiotics

C Women with spontaneous rupture of membranes at term of 18 hours duration routinely treated with antibiotics

D Women undergoing caesarean delivery should be administered with oral antibiotics following delivery

E Prophylactic antibiotics should be given to all women who had operative vaginal deliveries

6. **Regarding secondary prevention of preterm labour (PTL):**

A A positive oncofetal fibronectin test at 18 weeks of pregnancy is a strong predictor of PTL

B A positive fibronectin test is 100% predictive of PTL

C A woman with a negative fibronectin test and a cervical length of 30 mm should not be managed with tocolysis

D A woman with cervical length of < 25 mm at 28 weeks should be prescribed oral progesterone in lower resource countries

E A woman with a singleton pregnancy and a prior history of pre-term birth (PTB) with a short cervix at 24 weeks of pregnancy has an increased sensitivity of PTB of up to 40%

7. **Regarding cervical cerclage and preterm labour:**

A Cervical cerclage should be electively offered to women with a history of one mid-trimester pregnancy loss

B Cervical cerclage should be offered to women with no previous history of pre-term labour but who are noted to have a short cervix at 24 weeks

C Women with two previous miscarriages should be offered serial ultrasound assessment of cervix, and be offered cervical cerclage if cervical length is < 25 mm

D Perinatal mortality improves in women with twin pregnancies who have had an elective cerclage

E A rescue cervical cerclage at 24 weeks of pregnancy can delay delivery by an average of 10 weeks

8. **Regarding uultrasound scanning for fetal abnormalities:**

A Spina bifida can be detected during first trimester at 9 weeks of gestation by using transvaginal ultrasound scanning

B 'Lemon' and 'banana' signs are characteristic signs of neural tube defects

C 'Lemon' and 'banana' signs are detectable as early as 11 weeks of pregnancy

D Increased nuchal translucency is associated with chromosomal abnormalities

E Increased nuchal translucency is a predictor of intrauterine growth restriction

9. **An increased nuchal translucency is associated with which of the followings:**

A Down's syndrome

B Noonan syndrome

C Edwards' syndrome

D Cardiac defects

E Male fetuses

10. Regarding vasa praevia

  A   It is commonly diagnosed during second trimester

  B   It is usually diagnosed at birth and is largely asymptomatic

  C   It can lead to fetal hydrops

  D   It can be a direct cause of fetal death if not diagnosed antenatally

  E   Prenatal diagnosis can lead to improved perinatal outcome

11. Increased risk of aortic dissection during pregnancy is seen in the following condition:

  A   Edwards' syndrome

  B   Down's syndrome

  C   Marfan's syndrome

  D   Coarctation of aorta

  E   Bicuspid aortic valve

12. Regarding cardiac disease during pregnancy:

  A   If pregnant, women with a cardiac transplant should discontinue immunosuppressant treatment during first trimester

  B   Women with prosthetic metal mitral valve must continue taking warfarin throughout pregnancy

  C   The risk of embryopathy with warfarin treatment during the first trimester is 20% *5%.*

  D   There is a significant risk of fetal intracerebral bleeding when the mother has been on warfarin throughout pregnancy

  E   Peripartum cardiomyopathy usually presents in peripartum period and the woman has an underlying cardiac disease

13. Drugs to be avoided during breast-feeding:

  A   Acyclovir

  B   Low-dose aspirin

  C   Cephalosporins

  D   Clotrimazole

  E   Combined oral contraceptive pill

14. Drugs to be avoided during breast-feeding:

  A   Low molecular weight heparin

  B   Methyldopa

  C   Nifedipine

  D   Azothioprine

  E   Tetracycline

15. Regarding obstetric cholestasis

  A   It affects up to 5% of pregnancies   *0.5 — 2.0*

  B   There appears to be a genetic predisposition in a third of women

  C   It usually presents in 2nd trimester

  D   Initial symptoms are severe pruritus of the palms and soles of the feet

  E   Bile acid levels are usually normal

16. **Investigation of abnormal liver function tests in the 3rd trimester of pregnancy include:**
    A Plasma fibrinogen levels
    B Bile acid levels
    C Screening for hepatitis C and E
    D Screening for antismooth muscle antibodies
    E Screening for antimitochondrial antibodies

17. **In women with severe obstetric cholestasis and prolonged thrombin time the newborn is at increased risk of:**
    A Neonatal hypoxic encephalopathy
    B Neonatal hypobilirubinaemia
    C Meconium aspiration
    D Haemolytic anaemia
    E Intracranial haemorrhage

18. **The following risk factors are associated with acute fatty liver of pregnancy:**
    A Multiparity
    B Singleton pregnancy
    C Severe pre-eclampsia
    D Female fetus
    E Fetus is homozygous for fatty acid oxidation disorders

19. **The following statements about hepatitis B infection are correct:**
    A > 90% are asymptomatic
    B The course of acute hepatitis B is accelerated by pregnancy
    C Hepatitis B virus infection acquired in the 2nd trimester has a 90% chance of infecting the neonate
    D A positive serum surface antigen confirms high infectivity
    E Neonatal transmission rates are high irrespective of hepatitis E antigen load

20. **Regarding inflammatory bowel disease and pregnancy**
    A Ulcerative colitis affects any segment of bowel
    B Women tend to have increased flare ups during the 2nd and 3rd trimester
    C Active disease during pregnancy is a risk factor for intrauterine growth restriction
    D Women with inflammatory bowel disease are at increased risk of vitamin B12 deficiency
    E Treatment with sulfasalazine is contraindicated as it interferes with folic acid metabolism

21. **Which of the following is true for a twin pregnancy?**
    A Chorionicity cannot be reliably determined in the 1st trimester of pregnancy
    B Twin pregnancies cannot be dated accurately
    C Crown rump length (CRL) charts cannot be used to date twin pregnancies
    D A discrepancy in CRL measurement in twins is associated with fetal loss in 20% of cases
    E A discrepancy in CRL measurements in twins is highly suggestive of preterm delivery

Questions: SBAs

For each question, select the single best answer from the five options listed.

22. Which of the following is an indication for cervical length monitoring?

    A   Previous cervical surgery
    B   History of previous preterm delivery or mid-trimester loss
    C   Uterine anomaly such as a bicornuate uterus
    D   Previous termination of pregnancy
    E   Pre-term pre-labour rupture of membranes

23. Which of the following ultrasound Doppler velocity waveforms are used to monitor anti-D isoimmunisation?

    A   Middle cerebral artery
    B   Ductus venosus
    C   Uterine artery
    D   Umbilical artery
    E   Triscuspid

24. A 28-year-old woman recently diagnosed with primary tuberculosis is now pregnant on medication.

    Which of the following blood tests should be monitored?

    A   Liver function tests
    B   Urea and electrolytes
    C   Full blood count
    D   Drug levels
    E   C-reactive protein

25. A 32-year-old woman is 34 weeks pregnant and has been recently diagnosed with a chest infection.

    Which of the following organisms is the most likely cause?

    A   Influenza H1N1
    B   Chickenpox pneumonia
    C   Streptococcus pneumoniae
    D   Haemophilus influenzae type B
    E   Methicillin-resistant Staphylococcus aureus

26. A 25-year-old woman is 20 weeks pregnant and has a fall.

    What dose of anti-D is required to neutralise a 4 mL fetomaternal haemorrhage?

    A   250 IU
    B   500 IU
    C   1500 IU
    D   2000 IU
    E   1200 IU

27. A 39-year-old woman is 33 weeks pregnant and has been diagnosed with obstetric cholestasis.

    Which of the following is the best treatment option to manage the itching?

    A Chlorphenamine maleate
    B Corticosteroids
    C Emollients
    D Vitamin K
    E Uro-deoxycholic acid

28. A 25-year-old woman presents at 30 weeks' gestation with a 5-day history of headache, squint with 6th nerve palsy and papilledema. She is sent for a head CT which is normal.

    What is the most likely diagnosis?

    A Idiopathic intracranial hypertension
    B Pre-eclampsia
    C Trigeminal neuralgia
    D Migraine
    E Cerebral vein thrombosis

29. You see a 40-year-old primigravid woman in antenatal clinic at 37 weeks' gestation. The presentation is confirmed to be breech on ultrasound scan. She is very keen to have a normal vaginal delivery.

    Which of the following would you consider to be a high risk factor?

    A Small baby (< 2000 g)
    B High body mass index
    C Primiparity
    D Trisomy 18
    E Gestational diabetes

30. You are obtaining consent from a woman for elective caesarean section. She has had 3 previous caesarean sections.

    Which of the following is the most likely serious complication?

    A Bowel injury
    B Blood transfusion
    C Hysterectomy
    D Wound dehiscence
    E Bladder injury

31. A 20-year-old primiparous woman who was low risk at booking presents to the day unit for the first time at 34 weeks' gestation with a history of reduced fetal movements.

    Which of the following would be your management plan?

    A Refer for ultrasound scan
    B Admit for induction of labour

C If the cardiotocography is normal, discharge her

D Administer steroids

E Admit for observation

32. A 35-year-old woman presents 4 days after an emergency caesarean section for failure to progress. She is septic and has low blood pressure.

Which of the following is the most likely causative organism?

A Group A *Streptococcus*

B Group B *Streptococcus*

C *Escherichia coli*

D *Pseudomonas* spp.

E Methicillin-resistant *Staphylococcus aureus*

33. You are asked to see a 36-year-old woman on the postnatal ward who delivered a baby by forceps. She is complaining of paraesthesia over the medial aspect of her thigh and weakness on walking.

Which of the following nerves is most likely to have damaged?

A Femoral

B Ilioinguinal

C Lateral cutaneous of the thigh

D Obturator

E Sciatic

34. You are asked to see a 23-year-old woman on the postnatal ward because the midwives are concerned that she is behaving oddly.

Which of the following symptoms suggests puerperal psychosis?

A Bewildered and confused

B Mood swings from elation to sadness

C Irritability

D Tearful

E Tiredness or exhaustion

35. A 27-year-old woman is fully breast-feeding. What contraceptive advice would you give her?

A No need for contraception for 6/52

B Can start progesterone-only pill anytime

C Fully breast-feeding and amenorrhoeic for 12 months is 98% effective

D No combined oral contraceptive pill for 3 months

E Can have intrauterine contraceptive device after her 6-week check up

Questions: EMQs

Questions 36 – 38

Option list for Questions 36 – 38:

A Digital vaginal examination
B Ultrasound scan and digital vaginal examination
C Admit and observe
D Fetal fibronectin
E Sterile speculum examination
F High vaginal swab
G Ultrasound scan
H Amniocentesis
I Consider induction of labour
J Cardiotocography
K Admit for observation
L Commence erythromycin treatment for 10 days
M Full blood count and C-reactive protein check
N Discharge home with reassurance

For each description below, choose the single most appropriate management option from the above list of options. Each option may be used once, more than once, or not at all.

36. A 20-year-old primigravida presents to the day unit at 33 weeks' gestation with a history of leaking fluid per vaginum for the last few hours. Fetal movements are normal and there are no contractions felt.

37. A 32-year-old multigravida presents to the day unit following a sudden gush of clear fluid per vaginum at 32 weeks of gestation. Fetal movements are normal and there are no contractions felt. On examination the pad is dry and no leaking fluid can be visualised on speculum examination.

38. A 28-year-old woman in her second pregnancy who was low risk at booking comes in at 35 weeks of gestation with clear fluid visibly leaking per vagina. She has no contractions and cardiotocography is normal.

Questions 39 – 41

Option list for Questions 39 – 41:

A Attend the emergency department
B Varicella zoster immune globulin as soon as possible
C Discharge home with reassurance
D Oral acyclovir
E Intravenous acyclovir
F Amoxicillin and oral acyclovir
G Blood test to confirm varicella zoster immunity
H Careful history to determine significance and susceptibility to infection
I Notify general practitioner or midwife
J Admit and observe
K Consider hospital assessment

For each description below, choose the single most appropriate answer from the above list of options. Each option may be used once, more than once, or not at all.

39. A 32-year-old school teacher is 10 weeks pregnant in her first pregnancy and contacts her general practitioner because one of the children in her class has contracted chickenpox.

H

40. A 32-year-old woman in her first pregnancy is 11 weeks pregnant. She visits her general practitioner as she has come into contact with chickenpox 2 days ago. A serum test finds her to be non-immune.

B

41. A 28-year-old woman in her second pregnancy visits her general practitioner at 20 weeks as she has a rash on her legs. She saw her cousin a week ago, and her cousin's son had chickenpox.

K

Questions 42 – 44

Option list for Questions 42 – 44:

A	Induction of labour	G	Elective caesarean section is not recommended
B	Induction of labour is not recommended	H	Emergency caesarean section
C	Instrumental delivery	I	McRoberts' manoeuvre
D	Episiotomy	J	Rubin manoeuvre
E	Fundal pressure	K	Knee-chest position
F	Consider elective caesarean section	L	Fetal blood sampling

For each description below, choose the single most appropriate management option from the above list of options. Each option may be used once, more than once, or not at all.

42. A 34-year-old diabetic woman in her first pregnancy has a suspected large-for-gestational-age fetus. Ultrasound scan confirms fetal macrosomia with an estimated fetal weight of 4.5 kg. She is anxious to discuss the mode of delivery.

F

43. A 34-year-old woman in her second pregnancy has an ultrasound scan with an estimated fetal weight of 4.5 kg at 37 weeks. She is requesting an elective caesarean section.

G

44. A 34-year-old multiparous woman is in the second stage of labour at 42 weeks' gestation. Upon the delivery of head, it remains tightly applied to the vulva and retracts slightly with the contraction.

I

Questions 45 – 47

Option list for Questions 45 – 47:

A	Fundal pressure	G	Emergency caesarean section
B	Instrumental delivery	H	Vaginal delivery is contraindicated
C	Episiotomy	I	Augmentation of labour with syntocinon
D	Breech extraction		
E	External cephalic version	J	Epidural anaesthesia
F	Ultrasound scan to assess presentation	K	Fetal blood sampling from the buttocks

For each description below, choose the single most appropriate delivery option from the above list of options. Each option may be used once, more than once, or not at all.

45. A 35-year-old multiparous woman has opted for a vaginal breech delivery, following a previous successful vaginal breech delivery. She is now in the second stage of labour but there is a delay in the descent of the breech.

46. A 32-year-old multiparous woman, who has had a previous caesarean section, is found to have a breech presentation at 36 weeks' gestation. She is requesting a vaginal breech delivery.

47. A 29-year-old multiparous woman, having had three normal deliveries, presents at 39 weeks for an external cephalic version. On the cardiotocography she is found to be regularly contracting 3 in 10.

Questions 48 – 50

Option list for Question 48 – 50:

A	At 31 weeks	H	At 39 weeks
B	At 32 weeks	I	Weekly from 16 weeks
C	At 33 weeks	J	Weekly from 20 weeks
D	At 34 weeks	K	Fortnightly from 16 weeks
E	At 35 weeks	L	Fortnightly from 10 weeks
F	At 36–7 weeks	M	Fortnightly from 24 weeks
G	At 38 weeks		

For each description below, choose the single most appropriate timings from the above list of options. Each option may be used once, more than once, or not at all.

48. A 40-year-old primiparous woman has a scan at 9 weeks confirming monochorionic monoamniotic twins. She is now at 28 weeks' gestation and she wishes to discuss the timing of delivery.

49. A 32-year-old multiparous woman has a monochorionic twin pregnancy. The planning of antenatal follow up is being planned.

50. A 28-year-old woman has conceived monochorionic diamniotic twins via in-vitro fertilisation. She wants to know the plan for delivery.

Answers: MCQs

1. A False

    B False

    C True

    D False

    E True

    The risk of teenage maternal mortality rate is less than for women aged over 30 years. Infant mortality rate is 60% higher than background obstetric population. Teenage mothers are at increased risk of postpartum depression. Teenage mothers had higher risk of small-for-date babies. Because of poor nutrition, they are more likely to be folic-acid deficient, hence at increased risk of neural tube defects.

2. A False

    B False

    C False

    D True

    E True

    The increased risk of maternal sepsis is attributed to changing demographics; such as increased age at first pregnancy, obesity and insulin dependent diabetes but not hypothyroidism. Anaemia per se reduces resistance; therefore a major haemorrhage is a risk factor. Non-white Caucasians are at increased risk of maternal sepsis. The enhanced virulence of circulated group A *Streptococcus* has been postulated.

3. A False

    B False

    C True

    D False

    E False

    The UK Confidential Enquiries Report (2009–2012) has found about 2% of all group A *Streptococcus* infections manifest as puerperal sepsis and it is community acquired. It usually presents as a sore throat but progresses rapidly to life-threatening maternal sepsis. Most group A *Streptococcus* infection cases occur during postpartum period.

4. A False

    B False

    C True

    D False

    E False

A tachycardia (> 100 beats/min), respiratory rate (> 20 breaths/min) and a temperature either > 38°C or < 35°C are signs of septicaemic shock. Furthermore, hypotension (systolic blood pressure of 90 or below) and urine output < 0.5 mL/kg/hr are other signs.

5. A False

    B False

    C False

    D False

    D False

Oral erythromycin should be only given to women with confirmed pre-term rupture of membranes where high vaginal swab has been taken and further digital examinations are avoided. Women with group B *Streptococcus*-positive high vaginal swabs during pregnancy should not be treated as infection recurs. They should be treated with intravenous antibiotics during labour, especially if chorioamnionitis is suspected. Women with spontaneous rupture of membranes and without signs of infection and duration of < 24 hours should not be routinely given antibiotics. Women undergoing caesarean section should receive antibiotic prophylaxis before skin incision. There is no evidence to support that routine use of prophylactic antibiotics at operative vaginal birth reduces the risk of sepsis.

6. A False

    B False

    C True

    D True

    E False

Oncofetal fibronectin is a glycosylated glycoprotein found in plasma and extracellular matrix. It has been identified in the amniotic fluid, extracts of placental tissue and in the cervicovaginal secretions prior to 20–22 weeks. Testing during the first half of pregnancy is therefore unhelpful in the prediction of impending prevention of preterm labour (PTL).

A positive fibronectin test is associated with an increased risk of PTL in symptomatic patients and negative test is indicative of lower risk. The European Association of Perinatal Medicine has recommended that women with cervical length of > 25 mm and fibronectin negative test do not require initiation of tocolysis.

Cervical length of < 25 mm is a useful indicator if there is a previous history of PTL. Such women should be assessed from 14–24 weeks and cervical cerclage be offered up till 24 weeks.

For women at 28 weeks in low resource countries, the International Federation of Gynecology and Obstetrics (FIGO) recommends the use of oral progesterone as it reduces the relative risk of PTL relative to placebo (at 28, 33 and 35 weeks) by a relative risk of 0.50, 0.58 and 0.69.

Women with a short cervix at 24 weeks and a history of PTL have an increased sensitivity to 70% of PTL.

7. A False

B False

C True

D False

E False

Cervical cerclage offers no significant benefit to women with 2 or fewer pre-term labours. Women with a shortened cervix at ultrasound scan with previous history of preterm labour or preterm prelabour rupture of membranes are more suited for cervical cerclage. Women with multiple pregnancies, even in the presence of shortened cervix, do not seem to benefit from cerclage and there is even evidence of increased perinatal mortality by increased risk of preterm deliveries and miscarriages. A rescue cervical cerclage had an average delay of 4 weeks prior to delivery.

8. A True

B False

C False

D True

E False

Several reports have described the detection of spina bifida as early as 9 weeks. 'Lemon' and 'banana' signs are diagnostic markers are for spina bifida and become apparent only in early second trimester. Increased translucency is associated with an increased risk of aneuploidy. Increased nuchal translucency with normal chromosomes is associated with adverse neonatal outcomes but not with the risk of growth restriction.

9. A False

B True

C False

D True

E True

Increased nuchal translucency is a marker for chromosomal abnormalities and is also associated with a wide spectrum of structural anomalies (most commonly cardiac defects). Male fetuses tend to have a slightly bigger nuchal translucency compared to female fetuses. Noonan's syndrome is the most frequently reported genetic syndrome in association with increased nuchal translucency. It is an autosomal dominant disorder.

10. A False

   B False

   C False

   D False

   E True

   The classical presentation of vasa praevia is by painless vaginal bleeding following rupture of the membranes. The cardiotocographic tracing will show fetal distress or fetal death. Although not routinely screened antenatally, there are reports of improved perinatal outcomes where it was diagnosed antenatally.

11. A False

   B False

   C True

   D True

   E True

   Increased risk of aortic dissection is associated with Marfan's syndrome, Ehlers–Danlos syndrome type IV, bicuspid aortic valve, Turner's syndrome and coarctation of aorta.

12. A False

   B True

   C False

   D True

   E False

   Women with cardiac transplant should not discontinue their immunosuppressants. Women with metal mitral valve are at increased risk of emboli and it is preferable that they continue with warfarin especially if the dosage is <5 mg. There is a risk of embryopathy of 5%. Discussion should involve the cardiologist, to decide if she can be switched over to low molecular weight heparin to reduce the risk of fetal intracerebral bleeding.

   Peripartum cardiomyopathy is a pregnancy-specific condition presenting with heart failure secondary to left ventricular systolic dysfunction without any underlying cardiac lesion.

13. A False

   B False

   C True

   D False

   E True

Acyclovir for the treatment of herpes infection is safe. Low-dose aspirin is safe but high doses of aspirin should be avoided. Cephalosporins cause diarrhoea and thrush in the baby. Clotrimazole is safe as there is a poor oral viability and it is thus highly unlikely to adversely affect the breast-fed baby. Combined oral contraceptive pill contains oestrogens which may lower milk production. Progestogen-only pills are safe.

14. A False

   B False

   C False

   D True

   E True

Low molecular weight heparins are not expected to be excreted into breast milk. Methylodopa and nifedipine have a minimal risk to baby. Azothiaprine should be avoided when breast-feeding babies. Tetracyclines can affect teeth development.

15. A False

   B True

   C False

   D True

   E False

The true incidence of obstetric cholestasis is 0.5–2.0%. There appears to be a genetic predisposition in a number of women which is very much related to a genetic aberration of a biochemical nature. It usually presents in the 3rd trimester. Bile acids are always abnormal, and along with deranged levels in a liver function test, is a cornerstone for the diagnosis of cholestasis.

16. A False

   B True

   C True

   D True

   E True

Prothrombin time should be checked as vitamin K deficiency is present in obstetric cholestasis. Bile acid levels will be abnormal. Other etiologies such as hepatitis A, B, C and E should be screened for, and also to check for auto-immune diseases and viral illnesses.

17. A False

   B False

   C True

   D True

   E True

Patients with obstetric cholestasis will have vitamin K deficiency. They will have increased tendency to bleeding. Therefore, it is recommended that women should be treated with oral vitamin K antenatally prior to delivery. These women are at increased risk of postpartum haemorrhage. As the baby is vitamin K deficient, there is increased risk of haemorrhage related complications.

18. A False

    B False

    C True

    D False

    E True

The incidence of acute fatty liver of pregnancy ranges between 1:7,000 and 1:12,000 pregnancies. It commonly presents in the 3rd trimester. It affects nulliparous women with twin pregnancies, and pregnancies with male fetus are at increased risk. It is thought to be associated with heterogenicity for long chain 3-hydroxy-acyl-coenzyme A dehydrogenase deficiency. Acute fatty liver of pregnancy can also occur in women with this disorder if the fetus is homozygous for fatty acid oxidation disorder.

19. A True

    B False

    C False

    D False

    E False

The majority of women with hepatitis B infection are asymptomatic. The course of acute hepatitis B is not accelerated by pregnancy. The hepatitis B infection acquired in the 1st and 2nd trimesters is less infective compared to the one acquired in 3rd trimester. It is the estimation of E antigen which indicates high infectivity rather than serum surface antigen. The presence of hepatitis E antigen and a high hepatitis B viral load has infection rates of 80–90%, in contrast to 5–10% infectivity rates with hepatitis E antigen negative.

20. A False

    B False

    C True

    D True

    E False

Ulcerative colitis mainly affects the large bowel, whereas Crohn's disease can affect any part of the bowel. Pregnancy has no effect on natural history. Most often flares up occur in postpartum phase, especially among women with Crohn's disease. Active disease during pregnancy is a risk factor for intrauterine growth restriction and these mothers should be closely monitored with serial ultrasound scanning.

Women with inflammatory bowel disease are at increased risk of deficiency of vitamin B12, folic acid and iron which should be checked and supplements provided. Sulfasalazine is safe during pregnancy and can be given. It does interfere with folate metabolism. Therefore, a high dose of folic acid (5 mg daily) is recommended.

21. A False

   B False

   C False

   D False

   E False

   F False

Chorionicity is best determined during the 1st trimester using lambda and T signs. Twin pregnancies can be accurately dated in the 1st trimester using singleton crown-rump length (CRL) charts. There are no validated fetal growth charts for twins. There is no significant difference between the CRL of twins and singleton pregnancies during the 1st trimester. The data on fetal outcome around the discrepancy in CRL in early pregnancy is conflicting. It is not a good predictor of early pregnancy loss. Twin-to-twin transfusion syndrome is usually diagnosed in the 2nd trimester.

Answers: SBAs

22. B History of previous preterm delivery or mid-trimester loss

Without a history of cervical weakness, an incidental finding of a shortened cervix is not an indication of suture insertion.

23. A MCA

MCA Doppler at ultrasound is used to monitor isoimmunisation.

24. A Liver function tests

Liver function tests need to be monitored due to the treatment regime.

25. C *Streptococcus pneumoniae*

Streptococcus pneumoniae is the most common cause.

26. B 500 IU

500 IU will neutralise up to 4 mL of fetomaternal haemorrhage. For each mL thereafter 250 IU extra is required.

27. A Chlorphenamine maleate

Chlorphenamine maleate is the most effective way to manage the itchy symptoms.

28. E Cerebral vein thrombosis

The incidence of cerebral vein thrombosis is 1 in 10,000 and is associated with high mortality rates.

29. A Small baby (< 2000 g)

Unfavourable factors for vaginal breech delivery include extremes of weight (<2 kg or > 3.8 kg), previous caesarean and keeling or footling breech presentation.

30. E Bladder injury

There is a 1 in 100 risk of bladder injury.

31. C If the cardiotocography is normal, discharge her

The first line investigation would be a cardiotocography. As this is her first presentation with reduced fetal movements, if the cardiotocography is normal no further investigation is required.

32. A Group A *Streptococcus*

In the last triennium the most common cause of direct maternal deaths in the UK was sepsis mainly due to Group A *Streptococcus*.

33. A Femoral

The femoral nerve is most often damaged when the nerve is compressed against the pelvic side wall. It can occur in inappropriate positioning in lithotomy.

34. B Mood swings from elation to sadness

Postpartum psychosis is a severe mental illness with a dramatic onset shortly after childbirth.

35. B Can start progesterone-only pill anytime

The progesterone-only pill (POP) is suitable straight away for breast-feeding women. Lactational amenorrhoea alone is not sufficient.

Answers: EMQs

36. E Sterile speculum examination

A sterile speculum examination after history is the best way to diagnosis preterm prelabour rupture of membranes.

37. G Ultrasound scan

An ultrasound can be useful to confirm or refute the diagnosis of preterm prelabour rupture of membranes, when the diagnosis is unclear as may show oligohydramnios.

38. I Consider induction of labour

Delivery should be considered from 34 weeks if preterm prelabour rupture of membranes has occurred, the health of the mother is the primary indicator for delivery.

39. H Careful history to determine significance and susceptibility to infection

80–85% of adults have had chickenpox in childhood.

40. B Varicella zoster immune globulin as soon as possible

As she is seronegative she should be given VZIG as soon as possible, it can be given up to 10 days.

41. K Consider hospital assessment

Pregnant women are at higher risk of complications, including pneumonia and so should be thoroughly assessed.

42. F Consider elective caesarean section

Fetal macrosomia associated with diabetes is a risk factor for stillbirth and shoulder dystocia.

43. G Elective caesarean section is not recommended

The prenatal diagnosis of fetal macrosomia is imprecise and prophylactic caesarean and induction of labour has not been shown to reduce the rate of shoulder dystocia in non-diabetic patients.

44. I McRoberts' manoeuvre

McRoberts' manoeuvre is the single most successful intervention for shoulder dystocia.

45. G Emergency caesarean section

Failure of the presenting part to descend may suggest pelvic disproportion and caesarean delivery should be considered.

46. H Vaginal delivery is contraindicated

A previous caesarean section is a poor predictive factor for vaginal breech delivery.

47. F Ultrasound scan to assess presentation

External cephalic version can still be done if membranes are intact, but presentation should be confirmed first.

48. B At 32 weeks

Delivery at 32 weeks is recommended due to the risk of cord entanglement.

49. K Fortnightly from 16 weeks

Ultrasound is conducted between 16–24 weeks to detect twin-to-twin transfusion. After 24 weeks fetal growth restriction needs to be detected.

50. F At 36–37 weeks

There is a higher risk of fetal demise in twins, so delivery is recommended around 37 weeks.

Chapter 24

Mock paper 2: gynaecology

Question: MCQs

Answer each stem 'True' or 'False'.

1. A 70-year-old woman who has two children presents with a grade 2 cystocele which has been present for the past 2 years. Occasionally, this bulge causes difficulty in emptying her bladder and she has to digitally push it back to micturate. She wakes up occasionally at night to go to the toilet, maybe once or twice. She is not sexually active.

   What management options would you consider for this woman at her first visit to the clinic?
   - A Assess a midstream specimen of urine for culture and sensitivity
   - B Urodynamics investigations
   - C Pelvic floor muscle training
   - D Ring pessary insertion
   - E Advise pelvic floor repair

2. Vaginal hysterectomy as part of the treatment for pelvic floor prolapse is associated with:
   - A Reduced risk of urinary incontinence in future
   - B Reduced risk of subsequent prolapse of pelvic organs
   - C Improved quality of sexual life
   - D Reduced recurrent risk of apical vault prolapse
   - E Increased risk of repeat surgery for prolapse in future

3. Causes of premature ovarian failure are:
   - A Iatrogenic – familial
   - B Childhood cancer treatment with cyclophosphamide
   - C Childhood cancer treatment with cisplatin
   - D Kallman's syndrome
   - E Radiation treatment for Wilm's tumour

4. Causes of premature ovarian failure include:
   - A Auto-immune thyroiditis
   - B Addison's disease

✓C   Turner's syndrome
✓D   Fragile X syndrome
✓E   Genital tuberculosis

5.   **Causes of premature ovarian failure include:**
  A   Hypoprolactinaemia
  ✓B   Sheehan's syndrome
  ✓C   Hypoparathyroidism
  ✗D   Hypothyroidism
  E   Chronic renal failure

6.   **Regarding the conservation of fertility after gynaecological cancer diagnosis:**
  ✓A   Large cone biopsy is a recognised treatment for stage IA1 of cervical cancer
  B   Large loop electrosurgery is a recommended treatment of stage IA2 cervical cancer
  ✓C   Radical vaginal trachelectomy is a standard method for treatment of women with large stage IA2 tumours up to 1–2 cm
  D   An overall 5-year survival following fertility-sparing surgery for early-stage cancer of cervix is much better for squamous cell cancer than adenocarcinoma
  E   Following trachelectomy, this is no increased risk of preterm labour

7.   **Causes of hyperprolactinaemia include:**
  A   Acromegaly
  ✓B   Renal failure
  ✗C   Hyperthyroidism
  ✓D   Phlebotomy
  E   Premature ovarian failure

8.   **A 35-year-old nulliparous woman has presented with a complaint of heavy, irregular menstruation. Her ultrasound scan has shown the presence of a bulky uterus with a submucosal fibroid measuring 3 cm in diameter. She wishes to discuss her fertility conserving treatment options.**

  What management options would you consider for this woman?
  ✓A   Combined oral contraceptive
  B   Injectable progestogens
  C   Endometrial resection of fibroid
  D   Myomectomy
  ✓E   Ulipristal acetate

9.   **Recognised common side effects of medicines used for the treatment of heavy menstrual bleeding are:**
  A   Worsening of asthma associated with levonorgestrel-releasing intrauterine system
  ✗B   Weight gain associated with combined oral contraceptives
  ✓C   Indigestion associated with non-steroidal anti-inflammatory drugs
  ✓D   Endometrial thickening associated with ulipristal acetate
  E   Vertigo associated with gonadotrophin-releasing hormone analogue

10. **Possible unwanted outcomes following an intervention experienced by some women are described as following:**
    A   Common (1 in 200 chance)
    B   Less common (1 in 500 chance)
    C   Less common (1 in 1000 chance)
    D   Rare (1 in 5,000 chance)
    E   Very rare (1 in 100,000 chance)

11. **Regarding multiple pregnancies after assisted reproductive treatment:**
    A   There is no reduction in multiple pregnancies rate after two-embryo transfer compared with three-embryo transfer
    B   Single-embryo transfer leads to a cumulative pregnancy rate comparable to double embryo transfers
    C   Women carrying multiple pregnancies following assisted conception treatment have the same rates of complication compared to those conceiving spontaneously
    D   Ultrasound scanning in 2nd trimester for fetal abnormalities screening in twin pregnancies is less sensitive as compared with singleton pregnancies
    E   In screening for fetal growth in twin pregnancies, scanning should be carried out every 2 weeks from 20 weeks' gestation

12. **Regarding colposcopy examination**
    A   It allows visualisation of the abnormal areas within the cervical canal   TZ
    B   3% acetic acid application will stain cervical intraepithelial neoplasia (CIN) lesions as brown
    C   A green filter may be used for visualisation of vascular pattern
    D   Mosaicism and punctuations are classical patterns of CIN
    E   Columnar epithelium stains brown with Lugol's iodine

13. **A 40-year-old woman with dysfunction uterine bleeding has an endometrial biopsy. The histology showed endometrial hyperplasia. The risk factors for developing endometrial hyperplasia are:**
    A   Genetic predisposition   No genetic
    B   Unopposed progestogens
    C   Prolonged treatment with tamoxifen
    D   Theca cell tumours   ⎤ Androgen
    E   Sertoli Leydig cell tumours ⎦

14. **A 30-year-old woman presents with irregular and infrequent periods and had an endometrial biopsy. Upon physical examination there are virilising signs as well.**

    Which of the following are possible contributors?

    A   Obesity
    B   Polycystic ovarian disease
    C   Granulosa cell ovarian tumour
    D   Sertoli cell tumour
    E   Hilus cell tumour

15. **Which of the following are ultrasound features suggestive of benign cyst?**
    - A Smooth multilocular cyst with largest diameter of 100 mm
    - B Absence of acoustic shadows
    - C Unilocular cyst
    - D Irregular solid areas within a unilocular cyst
    - E At least two papillary structures within the cyst

16. **Regarding the adverse effects of chemotherapy for ovarian cancers:**
    - A Carboplatin is associated with alopecia
    - B Paclitaxel is associated with irreversible alopecia
    - C Carboplatin is associated with pancytopenia
    - D Cyclophosphamide is associated with neuropathy
    - E Cyclophosphamide is associated with haemorrhagic cystitis

17. **Adenomyosis can be diagnosed on ultrasound by the following features:**
    - A The presence of endometrial cystic areas located close to myometrial junction
    - B The presence of asymmetric myometrial walls
    - C Circular blood flow around the cystic areas
    - D The presence of round lesions
    - E The presence of diffusely scattered myometrial vascularity

18. **Which of the following contraceptive methods can be used by women living with HIV?**
    - A Combined oral contraceptives
    - B Progestogen only pill
    - C Depo medroxy progesterone
    - D Copper intrauterine device
    - E Levonorgestrel progestin only implants

19. **Regarding first trimester termination of pregnancy and intrauterine systems:**
    - A There is a 5% increased risk of infection
    - B The expulsion rate is approximately 10%
    - C There is a significantly higher rate of uterine perforation as compared to the non-pregnant stage
    - D It does not affect regularity of menstrual cycles
    - E Failure rates are the same irrespective of parity

20. **Combined oral contraceptives and health benefits:**
    - A Reduces the risk of osteoporosis
    - B Reduces the risk of carcinoma of the cervix
    - C Reduces the risk of breast cancer in women carrying the *BRCA2* mutation
    - D Reduces the risk of developing ovarian cancers well into menopause
    - E Reduces the risk of a tubal ectopic pregnancy

21. **A 42-year-old woman who has two children is being scanned at her booking visit and she is now 11 weeks pregnant. The sonographer suspects that it is a dichorionic twin pregnancy but is unable to carry out a nuchal translucency scan for one of the twins. Regarding this woman:**

  ✗ **A**   The twins must be dizygotic

  ✓ **B**   The risk of Down's syndrome is much higher in her age group than for a singleton pregnancy

  ✗ **C**   The risk of miscarriage following an amniocentesis test is about 5%

  ✗ **D**   The detection rate for Down's syndrome using the double test remains unaltered

  ✗ **E**   The chorionic villous sampling related pregnancy miscarriage risk is about 10%

Questions: SBAs

For each question, select the single best answer from the five options listed.

22. You are consenting a 29-year-old woman for uterine artery embolisation and she wishes to know the impact it will have on future pregnancies.

    A   There is a lower risk of miscarriage compared to following a myomectomy
    B   There is a higher chance of premature delivery following the procedure
    C   There is no impact on the mode of delivery
    D   There is an increased chance of sustaining a postpartum haemorrhage
    E   There is an increased likelihood of a small-for-gestational-age baby

23. You are about to fit a 28-year-old woman with a levonorgestrel-releasing intrauterine system.

What is the most common associated risk?

    A   Failure of contraception in 1% of cases
    B   Infection in 10% of cases
    C   Expulsion in 1% of cases
    D   Expulsion in 5% of cases
    E   Perforation in 3% of cases

24. A 60-year-old woman presents to the clinic following an episode of postmenopausal bleeding.

At what endometrial thickness would you perform an endometrial biopsy?

    A   2 mm
    B   3 mm
    C   4 mm
    D   5 mm
    E   6 mm

25. A 19-year-old woman presents with a history of dysmenorrhoea, which of the following is a risk factor?

    A   Multiparity
    B   Early menarche
    C   Irritable bowel syndrome
    D   Intramural fibroids
    E   Oligommenorrhoea

26. A 30-year-old woman presents with secondary amenorrhoea, which of the following would put her at risk of premature ovarian failure?

    A   Renal failure
    B   Hepatitis C
    C   Hypothyroidism
    D   Rheumatoid arthritis
    E   Lupus

27. A 22-year-old woman has a body mass index of 31 and has recently been diagnosed with polycystic ovarian syndrome.

What is she most at risk of developing in the future?

  A Hypertension
  B Thromboembolism
  C Cataracts
  D Cervical cancer
  E Dysmenorrhoea

28. A 28-year-old woman is being followed up for gestational trophoblastic disease. Her β-hCG levels have normalised within 6 weeks of treatment.

How long should she be followed up for?

  A 6 months from the date of uterine evacuation
  B 1 year from the date of uterine evacuation
  C 6 months from the normalisation of the β-hCG level
  D 1 year from the normalisation of the β-hCG level
  E No further follow up needed

29. A 20-year-old woman presents with new onset hirsutism. She has a normal body mass index and a normal pelvic ultrasound scan, however she has a very elevated testosterone level and a high dehydro-epiandrosterone sulphate level.

What is the most likely diagnosis?

  A Acromegaly
  B Polycystic ovary syndrome
  C Adrenal tumour
  D Cushing's syndrome
  E Prolactinoma

30. A 73-year-old woman has ovarian cancer. The tumour involves both ovaries and there is microscopic evidence of peritoneal metastasis outside the pelvis (maximum 2 cm in size).

What stage ovarian cancer is this?

  A IIc
  B IIIa
  C IIIb
  D IIIc
  E IV

31. A 25-year-old woman has a family history of ovarian cancer and is found to have a 4 cm simple cyst. Which of the following increases her risk of ovarian cancer?

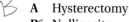

  A Hysterectomy
  B Nulliparity
  C Combined oral contraceptive pill use

    D Breast-feeding

    E Talcum powder use

32. In which of the following scenarios is it deemed safe to prescribe the combined oral contraceptive pill?

    A Body mass index greater than 40

    B Valvular heart disease with pulmonary hypertension

    C Benign liver tumours

    D Grandmother diagnosed with deep venous thrombosis

    E History of gestational trophoblastic disease and currently elevated β-hCG levels

33. During investigations for in vitro fertilisation, the husband is found to have a sperm count of < 20 million per mL on two separate occasions. Everything else is normal.

What is the most likely diagnosis?

    A Increased paternal age

    B Ejaculatory dysfunction

    C Congenital absence of the vas deferens

    D Varicocele

    E Primary testicular failure

34. A 36-year-old woman has been found to have a 5 cm intramural fibroid and an 8 cm submucosal fibroid.

Which of the following will reduce the size of the fibroids?

    A Mefanamic acid

    B Uterine artery embolisation

    C Hysterectomy

    D Progestogens

    E Endometrial ablation

35. An outpatient hysteroscopy is being performed for post-menopausal bleeding.

Which of the following is correct?

    A It is not suitable for nulliparous women

    B It can be performed via the vaginoscopic route

    C Polypectomies can only be performed under general anaesthetic

    D It should only be considered if there are contraindications to general anaesthesia

    E It is not suitable if the patient's body mass index is over 40

Questions: EMQs

Questions 36 – 40

Option list for Questions 36 – 40:

A	Admit and observe	H	Repeat serum β-hCG in 48 hours
B	Diagnostic laparoscopy and proceed	I	Laparoscopic salpingectomy
C	Trans-vaginal ultrasound scan and serum β-hCG	J	Fluid resuscitation
		K	Trans-vaginal ultrasound scan serum β-hCG and a chlamydia screen
D	Methotrexate		
E	Laparotomy and proceed	L	Progesterone level
F	Repeat trans-vaginal ultrasound scan	M	Fluid resuscitation followed by laparotomy
G	Repeat serum β-hCG in 24 hours		

For each description below, choose the single most appropriate management option from the above list of options. Each option may be used once, more than once, or not at all.

36. A 25-year-old woman has been diagnosed with an ectopic pregnancy on ultrasound scan. The mass has a heartbeat, there is no free fluid and the β-hCG is static at 5000 IU/L. She is haemodynamically stable and wishes to avoid surgery.

37. A 32-year-old woman has a positive pregnancy test and is at approximately 8 weeks' gestation. She presents due to vaginal spotting and pain on intercourse.

38. A 29-year-old woman is brought into the emergency department by ambulance after collapsing at work. She has a positive pregnancy test and an acute abdomen.

39. A 38-year-old multiparous woman attends for an early scan and is found to have an empty uterus. No mass is seen and there is no free fluid. She is haemodynamically stable. Her β-hCG today is 550 IU/L.

40. A 35-year-old multiparous woman, with an extensive surgical history has a known ectopic pregnancy. Her β-hCG has risen from 3000 IU/L to 3500 IU/L in 48 hours.

Questions 41 – 45

Option list for Questions 41 – 45:

A	Acute appendicitis	F	Tubo-ovarian abscess
B	Diverticulitis	G	Chlamydial infection
C	Pelvic endometriosis	H	Large fibroid uterus
D	Pelvic tuberculosis	I	Renal colic
E	Ovarian torsion		

For each description below, choose the single most appropriate diagnosis from the above list of options. Each option may be used once, more than once, or not at all.

41. A 19-year-old woman presents with history of sudden-onset lower abdominal pain worse in the left iliac fossa. She has felt nauseous but has not vomited. She is slightly tachycardic but otherwise haemodynamically stable. On abdominal examination there is some tenderness, guarding and rebound in the left iliac fossa. She cannot tolerate bimanual examination due to extreme tenderness.

42. A 14-year-old girl presents with a 12-hour history of severe abdominal pain, vomiting and fever. On examination she is tachycardic and there is presence of rebound tenderness and guarding in the lower abdomen.

43. A 35-year-old woman complains of severe dyspareunia, menorrhagia and dysmenorrhoea. On clinical examination there is tenderness in the pouch of Douglas.

44. A 50-year-old woman complains of abdominal pain for the past few months and long-term constipation. On examination she is tender, especially in the left lower abdomen.

45. A 25-year-old Asian woman presents with persistent pelvic pain. She has been in the UK for 2 years and gives a long history of lower abdominal pain, as well as painful sexual intercourse.

Questions 46 – 50

Option list for Questions 46 – 50:

A   Congenital adrenal hyperplasia
B   Premature thelarche
C   Premature pubarche/adrenarche
D   Central precocious puberty
E   Constitutional delay in growth and adolescence
F   Hypogonadotrophic hypogonadism
G   Klinefelter's syndrome
H   Turner's syndrome
I   Testicular feminisation syndrome

For each description below, choose the single most appropriate diagnosis from the above list of options. Each option may be used once, more than once, or not at all.

46. A 6-year-old girl is brought in by her parents who have noticed pubic hair development. On examination, she is on the 98th centile for height. She has stage 2 pubic hair development, stage 3 breast development and acne.

47. A 13-year-old girl is referred with short stature and delayed puberty. She suffers from asthma for which she requires additional salbutamol several times each week. On examination, she has pectus carinatum in keeping with long-standing asthma, but otherwise there is nothing of note. Her bone age is 10.5 years. Endocrine investigations show the following: estradiol 27 pmol/L, follicle-stimulating hormone 1.2 mU/L, luteinising hormone < 0.5 mU/L.

48. A 2-year-old girl is referred with a 6-month history of fluctuating breast development. Initially, the left breast was swollen. This subsided, but the right breast then became swollen, before resolving, only to recur again. She is otherwise well. Her mother says she is stubborn and difficult at times. On examination, she has modest stage 2 breast development on both sides, with the right being bigger than the left.

49. A 15-year-boy is referred with delayed puberty. He is healthy with no significant medical history, but had delayed speech and language development when younger. He is on the 91st centile for height. He has stage 2 pubic hair and testicular volumes of 2 mL. Preliminary investigations reveal the following: follicle-stimulating hormone 34.5 mU/L, luteinising hormone 23.6 mU/L, testosterone 1.1 nmol/L.

50. A 13-year-old girl was successfully treated for acute lymphoblastic leukaemia 5 years ago and attends for routine review. She had craniospinal irradiation and chemotherapy for 2 years. On examination, she is significantly overweight (> 99.6th centile), with a height on the 10th centile. There is possibly some early breast development, but in the context of the obesity it is difficult to be sure. There is no pubic hair. Investigations show follicle-stimulating hormone < 0.5 mU/L, luteinising hormone < 0.5 mU/L, estradiol < 18 pmol/L, prolactin 685 mU/L.

Answers: MCQs

1. A False

   B False

   C True

   D True

   E False

   This patient's history is not suggestive of cystitis or recurrent urinary tract infection. Urine should be routinely checked for nitrates and if positive then a sample should be sent away for culture and sensitivity. This patient did not complain of symptoms suggestive of detrusor instability (urgency, urgency incontinence, marked nocturia) therefore urodynamics investigations are not indicated. There is evidence to suggest that all women should be initially managed with conservative methods (pelvic floor exercises and ring pessary). Pelvic floor muscle training not only improves symptoms but anatomical defects of pelvic organ prolapse as well. Surgery should be reserved only for those where conservative management fails or they decline to accept pelvic floor exercises. The patient should be counselled about the risk of recurrence of prolapse.

2. A False

   B False

   C False

   D False

   E True

   It has been recognised that prolapse is purely a vaginal phenomenon and the uterus more or less acts as a deterrent. Vaginal hysterectomy done as part of POP repair is not a treatment of incontinence (which needs to be investigated and managed distinctly). Vaginal hysterectomy increases the risk of urinary symptoms, POP and apical vaginal vault thus requiring further surgery. Current opinion is to retain the uterus by using newer techniques rather than undertaking vaginal hysterectomy as part of pelvic floor repair. Furthermore it has been reported that occult urinary stress incontinence may become bothersome after anterior repair.

3. A True

   B True

   C False

   D False

   E True

   There is a familial tendency towards premature ovarian failure which is defined by certain chromosomal patterns. Childhood cancer treatment with cyclophosphamide does lead to irreversible ovarian damage but no such damage is seen with cisplatin. Kallman's syndrome is a cause of primary amenorrhoea but not premature ovarian failure. Radiation treatment for Wilm's tumour does involve radiation to the pelvis and it will knock out ovarian follicles. Patients with Turner's syndrome have an increased tendency towards premature ovarian failure, except the Turner's variant where patients do have some evidence of menstruation and then there is evidence of atrophic failure. Genital tuberculosis does lead to damage to the ovarian follicles. Any auto-immune disease such as thyroiditis or Addison's disease damages mature ovarian follicles but leaves primordial follicles intact. Sheehan's syndrome does lead to pan-hypopituitarism and that is the reason for premature ovarian failure. Hypothyroidism per se is not a cause of premature ovarian failure but could be part of the autoimmune phenomenon. Hypoprolactinaemia and hypoparathyroidism are types of pan-hypopituitarism and contribute to premature ovarian failure.

4. A True

 B True

 C True

 D True

 E True

See the answer to question 3.

5. A True

 B True

 C True

 D False

 E False

See the answer to question 3.

6. A True

 B False

 C True

 D False

 E False

The correct treatment is local excision along with pelvic lymph node dissection as there is a risk of lymph node involvement in < 5% with a 0.6% risk of parametrial involvement. Radical trachelectomy is a standard management of treatment for women with large stage IA2 and small stage IB1 tumours up to 2 cm, grade 1 and 2 and no lymphovascular invasion. An overall survival of 5 years is the same for both squamous and adenocarcinoma at early stage cervical cancer. Following trachelectomy there is an increased risk of mid trimester pregnancy loss (7%) and preterm delivery (10%) prior to 32 weeks.

7. A True

    B True

    C False

    D True

    E False

    Any pituitary tumour affecting function by overproduction of hormones that interferes with hypothalamo-pituitary axis will produce increased levels of prolactin. Any stress, even phlebotomy, can cause increased levels of prolactin. It is hypothyroidism but not hyperthyroidism associated with increased prolactin. Co-morbidities of renal failure explain increased levels of prolactin. Premature ovarian failure is diagnosed with raised levels of FSH and LH but will have lower levels of oestrogens and prolactin.

8. A True

    B False

    C False

    D False

    E True

    The combined oral contraceptive is an effective method of managing the majority of women provided there are no contraindications. Injectable progestogens have associated side effects and a higher chance of irregular cycles than treatment with the oral contraceptives.

    There is no evidence that endometrial ablation or myomectomy of sub mucosal fibroids will either improve the menstrual symptoms or enhance infertility.

    Ulipristal acetate is a new dynamic medicine for the treatment of fibroids. Data shows that women do not experience any oestrogens deficiency symptoms, become amenorrhoeic and fibroid size gradually decreases as well.

9. A False

    B False

    C True

    D True

    E False

    Indigestion and worsening of asthma is a side effect of non-steroidal anti-inflammatory drugs. Weight gain is a side effect of injectable progestogens, not of oral contraceptives. Endometrial thickening and vertigo are side effects of ulipristal acetate and not of gonadotrophin-releasing hormone analogue.

10. A False

    B False

C **True**

D **False**

E **True**

The correct figures are as follows:

- Common: 1 in 100 chance
- Less common: 1 in 1000 chance
- Rare: 1 in 10,000 chance
- Very rare: 1 in 100,000 chance

11. A **False**

B **True**

C **False**

D **False**

E **False**

Multiple pregnancy rates decline when two embryos are transferred as compared with transferring three embryos. Single-embryo transfer has not only led to reduced twins rates, but also a reduced pregnancy rates. However, cumulative pregnancy rates following single embryo transfer rates are as good as those achieved with two-embryo transfers.

Most women undergoing assisted reproductive techniques tend to have other underlying co-morbidities related to their average advanced at the time treatment, which statistically increase their risks of increased pregnancy-related complications as compared to those who conceive spontaneously.

Detection rates for fetal abnormalities in twins and triplets by ultrasound scanning are not significantly different to detection rates in singleton pregnancies.

Fetal growth assessment for monochorionic twins should start as early as possible but in dichorionic pregnancy, this should be more frequent as advised in NICE guidelines for dealing with multiple pregnancies.

12. A **False**

B **False**

C **True**

D **True**

E **False**

Colposcopy allows visualisation of the transformation zone and biopsies can be taken from the abnormal areas. Following acetic acid application, cervical intraepithelial neoplasia (CIN) lesions appear as aceto-white. Bizarrely, the appearance of blood vessels at green filter may suggest cancer. Intensity of mosaicism and punctuation are classical patterns for greater degrees of CIN. Columnar epithelium and immature metaplasia do not take up Lugol's iodine stain.

13. A **False**

   B **False**

   C **True**

   D **False**

   E **False**

There is no genetic predisposition for endometrial hyperplasia. Unopposed oestrogens treatment increases the risk of development of endometrial hyperplasia but not progestogens. Prolonged treatment with tamoxifen is associated with endometrial hyperplasia. Theca cell tumours and Sertoli-Leydig cell tumours are not oestrogen-producing tumours. They are in fact producers of androgenic hormones.

14. A **False**

   B **False**

   C **False**

   D **True**

   E **True**

Irregular and infrequent occurrence of periods and the associated virilising signs is suggestive of excess testosterone production in the body. Obesity will increase the risk of irregular periods but not because of virilisim. Women with polycystic ovarian cystic disease do suffer from irregular periods, but they do not exhibit signs of virilisation. Granulosa cell tumour is an oestrogen-producing tumour therefore cannot contribute towards virilisation. Virilisation is representative of abnormally high levels of testosterone. Sertoli cell tumours and hilus cell tumours are testosterone producing tumours.

15. A **True**

   B **False**

   C **True**

   D **False**

   E **True**

Features suggestive of malignancy are irregular, solid tumors with largest diameter >100 mm; at least four papillary structures; the presence of ascites; and a very strong blood flow.

Features of benign tumours are unilocular cysts; a solid component of < 7 mm; the presence of acoustic shadows; a smooth multilocular tumour, the largest diameter being < 100 mm; and no colour flow.

16. A **False**

   B **False**

   C **True**

D False

E True

Alopecia with carboplatin is a rare side effect. Alopecia associated with paclitaxel is reversible. Pancytopenia does occur with carboplatin and it is secondary to myelosuppresion, as is the case with cyclophosphamide. Neuropathy does not occur with cyclophosphamide but is a recognised complication of carboplatin. Patients on methotrexate can present with black stools, which is a serious side effect secondary to myelosuppresion.

17. **A** False

    B True

    C False

    D False

    E True

Adenomyosis foci are widely scattered in the myometrium and not in the endometrial cavity. Asymmetric myometrial walls are due to extensive fibrosis. Blood flow around adenomyosis is diffusely spread but not circular which is seen with fibroids. Round lesions are usually fibroids.

18. **A** True

    B True

    C True

    D False

    E False

Women living with HIV can use combined oral contraceptives, progestogens and injectable preparations. Intrauterine devices should be avoided.

19. **A** False

    B False

    C False

    D False

    E True

Large randomised trials and a Cochrane review have reported a low incidence of infection, uterine perforation and expulsion (1–2 per 100 women) whether an intrauterine contraceptive device (IUCD) is inserted immediately following surgical termination of pregnancy or an IUCD is inserted in a non-pregnant uterus several weeks following the termination of a pregnancy. More women on copper intrauterine system report a longer menstrual cycle as compared to those using a levonorgestrel-releasing intrauterine system. Failure rates are not influenced by parity.

20. A **False**

   B **False**

   C **False**

   D **True**

   E **True**

Combined oral contraceptive (COC) in perimenopausal hypoestrogenic women protects bone but there is no data on whether the rate of osteoporosis-related fractures is reduced. Over 5 years, there is an increased risk of cervical cancer and prolonged use also increases risk of breast cancer irrespective of *BRCA* gene status. COC does reduce the risk of developing ovarian cancer and this effect persists for several years after menopause. Compared with the use of an intrauterine device, there is a definitive reduction in the risk of ectopic pregnancy because of effective anovulation.

21. A **False**

   B **True**

   C **False**

   D **False**

   E **False**

A proportion of dichorionic twins are monozygous, although most are dizygous. The risk of miscarriage is doubled (around 2%) for both amniocentesis and chorionic villous sampling. The risk of at least one of the twins being affected is double the normal age related risk (1 in 80 plus 1 in 80). The detection rate of the combined test falls to 40–50% because of the dilution effect.

Answers: SBAs

22. D There is an increased chance of sustaining a postpartum haemorrhage

There is an increased risk of postpartum haemorrhage after uterine artery embolisation. Uterine artery embolisation also increases the risk of miscarriage compared to laparoscopic myomectomy.

23. D Expulsion in 5% of cases

The risk of expulsion is 5%, most frequently occurring in the first few months. The risk of perforation is uncommon (< 1 in 1000).

24. D 5 mm

When 5 mm is used as the cut-off point, sensitivity for detecting endometrial cancer is 96% with a 39% false positive rate.

25. B Early menarche

Risk factors for dysmenorrhoea include family history, smoking, nulliparity and early menarche.

26. C Hypothyroidism

13.8% of women with premature ovarian failure have hypothyroidism and 1.7% have insulin-dependent diabetes mellitus.

27. A Hypertension

Polycystic ovarian syndrome results in an increased risk of hypertension, dyslipidaemia, impaired glucose tolerance and hyperinsulinaemia.

28. A 6 months from the date of uterine evacuation

If β-hCG levels are normal within 56 days of the pregnancy event, then follow up is for 6 months from the date of evacuation, if not, it is for 6 months following the date of β-hCG normalisation.

29. C Adrenal tumour

Very high testosterone levels increase the chance of malignancy, and raised dehydroepiandrosterone is associated with an adrenal cause.

30. C 3b

See **Table 20.1**.

31. B Nulliparity

Ovulation is considered a risk factor, and a nulliparous woman will have a higher rate of ovulation compared to a parous woman or a nullipara on contraceptive pill. The risk of ovarian cancer is decreased by oral contraceptive use, breast-feeding, tubal ligation or hysterectomy and a history of pregnancy.

32. D Grandmother diagnosed with deep venous thrombosis

Family history in a first degree relative under 45 years old is a UKMEC category 3.

33. C Congenital absence of the vas deferens

Azoospermia and normal hormone levels are suggestive of an obstructive cause.

34. B Uterine artery embolisation

Uterine artery embolisation shrinks fibroids by approximately 50%.

35. B It can be performed via the vaginoscopic route

This no-touch approach is associated with less pain.

Answers: EMQs

---

36. I Laparoscopic salpingectomy

Although this patient wishes to avoid surgery, she does not fulfil the criteria for methotrexate as she has a live ectopic pregnancy.

---

37. K Trans-vaginal ultrasound scan serum β-hCG and a chlamydia screen

She should attend the early pregnancy assessment unit to rule out miscarriage or ectopic. All patients should have an β-hCG test, an ultrasound scan and a chlamydia screen.

---

38. M Fluid resuscitation followed by laparotomy

The patient is unstable and therefore requires urgent surgery to stop the bleeding, which is most likely from a ruptured ectopic pregnancy.

---

39. H Repeat serum β-hCG in 48 hours

She should have a repeat β-hCG as the level is below the discriminatory level and she is stable.

---

40. F Repeat trans-vaginal ultrasound scan

Due to the previous abdominal surgery, it would be prudent to see rescan and assess whether the patient is suitable for methotrexate.

---

41. E Ovarian torsion

The sudden onset nature and extreme tenderness on bimanual examination are suggestive of ovarian torsion.

---

42. A Acute appendicitis

The vomiting and fever along with rebound tenderness make acute appendicitis the most likely diagnosis here.

---

43. C Pelvic endometriosis

Menorrhagia, dysmenorrhoea and dyspareunia are the hallmark features of endometriosis.

44. B Diverticulitis

Given the patient's age and history of constipation, diverticulitis is most likely the cause of her pain.

45. D Pelvic tuberculosis

Pelvic tuberculosis can present with such features, and given the long-term nature of her pain and her move to the UK 2 years ago from a country with a high prevalence of tuberculosis, this is the best option from the list.

46. D Central precocious puberty

Central precocious puberty is defined as the onset of puberty at < 8 years in girls and < 9 years in boys. The patient is exhibiting normal pubertal changes prematurely.

47. E Constitutional delay in growth and adolescence

It is likely that steroid use has caused a constitutional delay in this girl's growth.

48. B Premature thelarche

Breast development any time from birth to 6 years of age is termed premature thelarche.

49. G Klinefelter's syndrome

The tall stature, small testicular volume and hormone profile is suggestive of Klinefelter's syndrome (XXY).

50. F Hypogonadotrophic hypogonadism

She is likely to have developed hypogonadotrophic hypogonadism as a result of her treatment for acute lymphoblastic leukaemia.

Further reading

Advisory Committee on Immunization Practices Workgroup on the Use of Vaccines during Pregnancy and Breastfeeding. Guiding principles for development of ACIP recommendations for vaccination during pregnancy and breastfeeding. Atlanta, Georgia: Advisory Committee on Immunization Practices; 2008.

Balen AH, Creighton SM, Davies MC, MacDougall J, Stanhope R. Paediatric and Adolescent Gynaecology – a multidisciplinary approach. Cambridge: Cambridge University Press; 2004.

Bhide A. Ultrasound in prenatal diagnosis. Best Pract Res Clin Obs Gynaecol 2014; 28: 429–442.

British Association for Sexual health and HIV. UK National Guideline for the management of pelvic inflammatory disease. Macclesfield: British Association for Sexual health and HIV, 2011.

British Medical Association and Royal Pharmaceutical Society. British National Formulary (71st edn). London: Br Med J Publishing Group; 2016.

Brosens I, Gordon A, Campo R, Gordts S. Bowel injury in gynaecologic laparoscopy. J Am Assoc Gynecol Laparosc 2003; 10:9–13.

Chapron C, Querleu D, Bruhat M, et al. Surgical complications of diagnostic and operative gynaecological laparoscopy: a series of 29,966 cases. Hum Reprod 1998; 13:867–872.

Domchek, SM, Friebel TM, Neuhausen SL, et al. Mortality after bilateral salpingo-oophorectomy in BRCA1 and BRCA2 mutation carriers: a prospective cohort study. Lancet Oncol 2006; 7:223–229.

Eppsteiner E, Boardman L, Stokedale CK. Vulvodynia. Best Pract Res Clin Obstet Gynaecol 2014; 28:1000–1012.

Faculty of Sexual and Reproductive Healthcare of the Royal College of Obstetricians and Gynaecologists. UK Medical Eligibility Criteria for Contraceptive Use (UKMEC). London: Faculty of Sexual and Reproductive Healthcare of the Royal College of Obstetricians and Gynaecologists; 2016.

Faculty of Sexual and Reproductive Health Clinical Effectiveness Unit. CEU guidance: drug interactions with hormonal contraception. London: Faculty of Sexual and Reproductive Health; 2012.

Gopal G, Haoura E, Mahmood T. Pruritus Vulvae. Obstetrics, Gynaecology and Reproductive Medicine 2016; 26:05–100.

Jansen FW, Kapiteyn K, Trimbos-Kemper TC, Hermans J, Trimbos JB. Complications of laparoscopy: a prospective multicentre observational study. Br J Obstet Gynaecol 1997; 104:595–600.

Kauff ND, Domchek SM, Friebel TM, et al. Risk-reducing salpingo-oophorectomy for the prevention of BRCA1 and BRCA2-associated breast and gynecologic cancer: a multicenter, prospective study. J Clin Oncol 2008; 26:1331–1337.

Kingston H. ABC of Clinical Genetics, 3rd edn. New Jersey: Wiley-Blackwell 2002.

Lobo RA, Davis SR, De Villiers TJ, et al. Prevention of diseases after menospause. Climacteric 2014; 17:540–556.

Maher C, Feiner B, Baessler K, et al. Surgical management of pelvic organ prolapse in women. Cochrane Database Syst Rev 2016; 30:CD004014.

Moyal-Barracco M, Wendling J. Vulvar Dermatosis. Best Pract Res Clin Obstet Gynaecol 2014; 28:946–958.

McPherson K, Metcalfe MA, Herbert A, et al. Severe complications of hysterectomy: the VALUE study. BJOG 2004; 111:688–694.

National Institute of Care Excellence. Heavy menstrual bleeding: assessment and management. Clinical guideline [CG44]. Manchester: National Institute of Clinical Excellence; 2007.

National Institute of Care Excellence. Headaches in over 12s: diagnosis and management. Clinical guideline [CG150]. Manchester: National Institute of Care Excellence; 2012.

National Institute of Care Excellence. Preterm labour and birth. NICE Guideline 25. Manchester: National Institute of Clinical Excellence; 2015.

Nelson-Piercy C. Handbook of Obstetric Medicine. Boca Raton, Florida: CRC Press; 2015.

Ng EHY, Ho PC. Sub fertility - current concepts in management. Best Prac Res Clin Obs Gynaecol 2012; 26:729–863.

O'Connor M, Nair M, Kurinczuk JJ, Knight M. UK Obstetric Surveillance System annual report 2016. Oxford: National Perinatal Epidemiology Unit; 2016.

Olson AL, Smith VJ, Bergstrom AO, et al. Epidemiology of surgically managed pelvic organ prolapse and urinary incontinence. Obstet Gynaecol 1997; 89:501–506.

O'Niel S, Eden J. The pathophysiology of menopausal symptoms. Obstet Gynaecol Reprod Med 2014; 24:349–356.

Qureshi H, Massey E, Kirwan D, et al. BCSH guideline for the use of anti-D immunoglobulin for the prevention of haemolytic disease of the fetus and newborn. Tranfusion Med 2014; 24:8–20.

Risch HA, McLaughlin JR, Cole DE. Prevalence and penetrance of germline BRCA1 and BRCA2 mutations in a population series of 649 women with ovarian cancer. Am J Hum Genetics 2001; 68:700-710.

Royal College of Obstetricians and Gynaecologists, Green-top Guidelines. London: RCOG. www.rcog.org.uk/guidelines.

Schmeler KM, Lynch HT, Chen L, et al. Prophylactic surgery to reduce the risk of gynecologic cancers in the Lynch syndrome. N Engl J Med 2006; 354:261–269.

Sherrard J, Donders G, White D. European (IUSTI/WHO) Guideline on the management of vaginal discharge. Int J STD AIDS 2011; 22:421--429.

Shaw RW, Luesley D, Monga AK. Gynaecology (4th edn). London: Churchill Livingstone; 2011.

Timmerman D, Valentin L, Bourne TH, et al. Terms, definitions and measurements to describe the sonographic features of adnexal tumours: a consensus opinion from the international Ovarian Tumour Analysis (IOTA) Group. Ultrasound Obstet Gynecol 2000; 16:500–505.

Tobias ES, Connor M, Ferguson-Smith M. Essential Medical Genetics, 6th edn. New Jersey: Wiley-Blackwell; 2011.

Trutnovsky G, Kamisan Atan I, Martin A, Dietz HP. Delivery mode and pelvic organ prolapse: a retrospective observational study. BJOG 2016; 123:1551–1556.

Valentin L. Imaging in Gynaecology. Best Prac Res Clin Obs Gynaecol 2014; 28:619.

van der Spuy Z. Challenges in fertility regulation. Best Prac Res Clin Obs Gynaecol 2014; 28:793-794.

Wellings K, Hutchinson C, Guthrie K, Baker PN. Teenage pregnancy. London: Royal College of Obstetricians and Gynaecologists; 2007.